DIABETES IN PRACTICE

Case Studies with Commentary

Boris Draznin, MD, PhD,
Editor

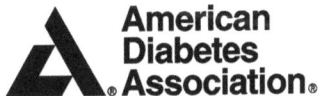

American Diabetes Association®

Director, Book Publishing, Victor Van Beuren; *Managing Editor*, John Clark; *Associate Director, Book Marketing*, Annette Reape; *Copyeditor*, Wendy Martin-Shuma; *Production Services*, Absolute Service, Inc.; *Printer*, Versa Press.

Printed in the United States of America
1 3 5 7 9 10 8 6 4 2

The suggestions and information contained in this publication are generally consistent with the *Standards of Medical Care in Diabetes* and other policies of the American Diabetes Association, but they do not represent the policy or position of the Association or any of its boards or committees. Reasonable steps have been taken to ensure the accuracy of the information presented. However, the American Diabetes Association cannot ensure the safety or efficacy of any product or service described in this publication. Individuals are advised to consult a physician or other appropriate health care professional before undertaking any diet or exercise program or taking any medication referred to in this publication. Professionals must use and apply their own professional judgment, experience, and training and should not rely solely on the information contained in this publication before prescribing any diet, exercise, or medication. The American Diabetes Association—its officers, directors, employees, volunteers, and members— assumes no responsibility or liability for personal or other injury, loss, or damage that may result from the suggestions or information in this publication.

∞ The paper in this publication meets the requirements of the ANSI Standard Z39.48-1992 (permanence of paper).

ADA titles may be purchased for business or promotional use or for special sales. To purchase more than 50 copies of this book at a discount, or for custom editions of this book with your logo, contact the American Diabetes Association at the address below or at booksales@diabetes.org.

American Diabetes Association
2451 Crystal Dr, Suite 900
Arlington, Virginia 22202

DOI: 10.2337/9781580407663

Library of Congress Control Number: 2021942304

Table of Contents

Preface

Over millennia, sharing the practical experience of one physician with others has been a proven way of disseminating best practices of the time with esteemed colleagues and teaching new generations of doctors. This selfless and generous sharing of knowledge is the cornerstone of teaching medical students and residents at the bedside and in classrooms, at local grand rounds and national conferences. The best way of acquiring clinical skills is to observe experienced physicians and to follow their example. Thus, learning from colleagues' experience is a time-tested learning process.

This book sets out to accomplish exactly that—to facilitate the learning process by sharing unusual and interesting cases with a great number of readers. We are fully aware that the readers may have had or currently have similar cases in their own practice and have selected similar or different approaches to their cases. Regardless, good clinicians always learn from others, always sharpen their own thought process, and always improve their acumen and skills.

Within these pages, you will find a compilation of 49 interesting cases from various fields of diabetology followed by short editorial commentaries to emphasize the major "take home" points of each case. I wish to thank Drs. Mary Korytkowski from the University of Pittsburgh, Louis Phillipson from the University of Chicago, and Anne Peters from the University of Southern California for their editorial help and commentary. Their opinions were of great value to me and I am certain will be of tremendous help and value to readers.

I also wish to thank all senior physicians and fellows in training for bringing their interesting cases to our attention and sharing with us their thought processes in terms of diagnosis and management of these cases. This is exactly what makes this book so interesting!

Finally, I wish to thank the American Diabetes Association's acquisition, publishing, and editorial staff for recognizing the need for this book and for helping us every step of the way to bring this book to light.

My outstanding agent, Ms. Joan Parker, deserves a special "Hooray"!

Boris Draznin, MD, PhD
The Celeste and Jack Grynberg Professor of Medicine
University of Colorado School of Medicine

Part 1

Atypical Diabetes

Case 1

Suspected Maturity-Onset Diabetes of the Young (MODY)-5 (MODY-HNF1B) Responding to Monotherapy With Metformin

Ana Ramirez Berlioz, MD[1] Richa Patel, MD[1] David Gardner, MD[1]
L. Romayne Kurukulasuriya, MD[1] and James Sowers, MD[1]

A thinly built 40-year-old Caucasian man with a past medical history of weight loss, polyuria, and polydipsia was admitted with sudden-onset mild epigastric pain, nausea, dizziness, lightheadedness, and excessive thirst. He also had hyperglycemia, hyponatremia, and elevated transaminases and serum creatinine. Hyperglycemia and hyponatremia resolved after intravenous (IV) hydration and IV insulin. However, he had persistently elevated creatinine and abnormal liver function tests upon discharge the following day and was instructed to establish care with Endocrinology.

On presentation to the Endocrinology clinic 1 week later, HbA$_{1c}$ (A1C) was elevated at 11%. He brought records of fasting glycemia with values ranging between 173 and 259 mg/dL. He was started on monotherapy with metformin extended release 500 mg daily, with instructions to increase dosing to twice a day after 1 week if tolerated. Based on the patient's body habitus, presentation, and response to therapy, latent autoimmune diabetes in adults (LADA) was suspected. GAD65 antibody, islet cell antibodies, and insulin antibodies were negative. Given his persistently elevated creatinine, a renal ultrasound was ordered, which disclosed left renal agenesis. At this point, it was noted that the patient's mother also had renal agenesis and had undergone a renal transplant.

The findings of diabetes, renal agenesis, and liver dysfunction in the setting of patient's family history were suggestive of monogenic diabetes, most likely maturity-onset diabetes of the young (MODY)-5 (MODY-HNF1B). Genetic testing performed at the University of Chicago has heterozygous whole gene deletion (Ch17:36,047,185–36,105,485) of HNF1B.

Patient continued monotherapy with metformin extended release 500 mg p.o. daily, with excellent glycemic control and stable renal function. His A1C dropped to 5.6% within 3 months of presentation and has remained stable since. He has established care with Nephrology and Hepatology. Further workup revealed elevated uric acid level and hypomagnesemia.

[1]Department of Medicine, Division of Endocrinology, Diabetes and Metabolism, University of Missouri–Columbia, Columbia, Missouri.

DOI: 10.2337/9781580407663.01

Diabetes is frequently classified as either type 1, characterized by autoimmune-mediated β-cell destruction and thus absolute insulin deficiency, or type 2, defined by progressive, relative insulin deficiency and associated insulin resistance. Both conditions are the result of complex polygenic and environmental factors. A lesser known and often misdiagnosed category known as MODY is represented by single-gene mutations. Assigning a patient a "type of diabetes" depends on the clinical and biochemical information available at the time of his or her presentation; however, some individuals will not fall clearly into a single category.[1] In the case of our patient, his body habitus pointed away from type 2 diabetes, but the absence of diabetic ketoacidosis on presentation and certainly his negative antibody panel were not suggestive of type 1 diabetes.

MODY is estimated to make up 1% of all cases of diabetes. Genetic mutations in 13 genes have been known to cause MODY through pancreatic β-cell dysfunction leading to hyperglycemia.[2] The three most common mutations are found in HNF4A, GCK, and HNF1A, making up the majority of all MODY cases.

HNF1B (hepatocyte nucleotide factor 1B) belongs to the homeobox-containing family of transcription factors and plays a central role in the development of the pancreas, kidneys, and liver. Over 50 different mutations have been reported within the HNF1B gene, located on chromosome 17q12. The most common of these is a whole gene deletion, which occurs in 50% of patients with MODY-HNF1B, also known as the 17q12 deletion syndrome. Patients with mutations in HNF1B (MODY-5) will almost always present with renal developmental disorders, especially renal cysts and renal dysplasia; they may additionally have genitourinary developmental anomalies, hyperuricemia, gout, abnormal liver function tests, and neurologic abnormalities, including developmental and speech delays, autism spectrum disorder, and schizophrenia.[3] These patients, unlike those with other MODY mutations, are not sensitive to sulfonylureas and thus will likely require exogenous insulin treatment.[4]

Establishing the diagnosis of MODY and distinguishing it from other forms of diabetes is challenging. This challenge exists partly because of provider unfamiliarity with this condition and a steadfast desire to classify patients into the more well-known type 1 versus type 2 categories, and in part because of limited access to genetic testing. However, it is important to try to identify MODY as a cause of diabetes, since once diagnosis is made, it allows for targeted treatment based on each affected gene.

COMMENTARY

This case is an interesting study describing the effectiveness of metformin in a patient with MODY-5, now classified as MODY-HNF1B. HNF1B is usually an insulin-deficit disorder and may not respond much to metformin or sulfonylurea preparations. Metformin addresses insulin resistance, which is not a hallmark of HNF1B. The most effective treatment for MODY-HNF1B is insulin and possibly glucagon-like peptide-1 receptor agonist (GLP-1RA) if enough cases can be accumulated to generate some data. Nevertheless, in this case, the patient responded well to metformin and remained stable throughout observation and follow-up.

Louis H. Philipson, MD, PhD, and Boris Draznin, MD, PhD

REFERENCES

1. American Diabetes Association. Classification and diagnosis of diabetes. *Diabetes Care* 2015;38(Suppl.):S8–S16

2. Anık A, Çatlı G, Abacı A, Böber E. Maturity-onset diabetes of the young (MODY): an update. *J Pediatr Endocrinol Metab* 2015;28:251–263. doi:10.1515/jpem-2014-0384

3. Roehlen N, Hilger H, Stock F, et al. 17q12 Deletion syndrome as a rare cause for diabetes mellitus type MODY5. *J Clini Endocrinol Metab* 2018;103:3601–3610. doi.org/10.1210/jc.2018-00955

4. Hattersley A, Bruining J, Shield J, Njolstad P, Donaghue KC. The diagnosis and management of monogenic diabetes in children and adolescents. *Pediatr Diabetes* 2009;10:33–42. doi.org/10.1111/j.1399-5448.2009.00571.x

Case 2

Maturity-Onset Diabetes of the Young (MODY)-4 Presenting as Gestational Diabetes

Ivana Sheu, MD,[1] Yung-In Choi, MD,[1] Samar Singh, MD,[1] and Ping H. Wang, MD[1]

A healthy 32-year-old Asian female with a strong maternal family history of diabetes was diagnosed with gestational diabetes on a routine pregnancy screening. She was started on insulin without complications during her pregnancy and remained euglycemic off of insulin after the birth of her first child. A few years later, the patient became pregnant with her second child without recurrent gestational diabetes. However, her pregnancy was complicated by premature rupture of membranes at week 34, requiring bed rest and antibiotics.

After the birth of her second child, the patient did not follow up because of a busy work schedule. At around 40 years old, she decided to reestablish care and, at that time, was diagnosed with presumed type 2 diabetes. Over the next 10 years, she was followed by an endocrinologist and tried multiple medications including metformin, exenatide, and sitagliptin, with medication intolerance due to nausea and abdominal discomfort. The patient was transitioned to insulin therapy. Given the patient's strong family history and gestational diabetes history, she was offered genetic testing and tested positive for a heterozygous IPF1 mutation (c.784C>A [p.Pro262Thr]) consistent with maturity-onset diabetes of the young (MODY)-4.

Currently, the patient is 59 years old with a BMI of 21.4 kg/m² and is on the Medtronic 670G insulin pump for labile blood glucose levels. Her most recent HbA_{1c} was 6.4% without hypoglycemia and with undetectable C-peptide levels. It is unclear if islet cell autoantibodies were obtained in the past. The patient's diabetes-related complications include mild autonomic and peripheral neuropathy, mild gastroparesis, and premature cataracts status post-extraction, with no evidence of diabetic kidney disease or retinopathy.

MODY is a rare group of autosomal-dominant diseases accounting for 1–2% of all diabetes diagnoses. Patients are often diagnosed with diabetes before the age of 25 years with atypical presentation of diabetes, strong family history of early-onset diabetes, and a prolonged honeymoon period before becoming insulin dependent. Here we will focus our discussion on MODY-4 as presented in our case.

---

[1]University of California Irvine Diabetes Center and Department of Medicine, Irvine, California.

DOI: 10.2337/9781580407663.02

5

MODY-4, first described by Stoffers et al. in 1997,[1] accounts for ~1% of all MODY diagnoses and is associated with a heterozygous insulin promoter factor-1 (IPF1) gene mutation. IPF1, also known as STF1, IDX1, and PDX1, is a homeodomain-containing protein that functions as a critically important transcription factor in pancreatic development and maintenance. IPF1 regulates islet cell apoptosis and hyperplasia through transcription regulation of downstream genes responsible for glucose sensing and insulin production, suppression of proapoptotic genes in islet cells, and endoplasmic reticulum folding and function. Similar defects in endocrine pancreas regulation have been seen in variations of IPF1 mutation outside of MODY-4 in other types of MODY and type 2 diabetes. In settings of homozygous IPF1 mutation, there have been reports of defects in pancreatic development and differentiation leading to neonatal pancreatic agenesis.

The presentation of MODY-4 differs from most other forms of MODY, with a later age of diabetes diagnosis averaging around 35 years old and a range of 13–67 years old. Also, the Michigan-Kentucky MODY-4 family pedigree study by Fajans et al.[2] described the presentation of obesity and hyperinsulinemia in some MODY-4 patients. Obesity is not a commonly associated finding with forms of MODY; however, there have been sporadic cases reported of obese patients with MODY-1, MODY-3, or MODY-6.

Once the diagnosis of MODY-4 has been made, most patients are able to achieve good glycemic control with lifestyle modifications or oral antihyperglycemic agents (often insulin secretagogues). A small number of patients require insulin at time of diagnosis. However, given the rarity of MODY-4, there have been limited reports of treatment strategies and long-term diabetes progression. There are two in detailed reports of MODY-4 with documentation of diabetes progression and management from China.[3,4] The patients were diagnosed with diabetes at the ages of 13 and 23 years; both were first initiated on insulin and then later transitioned to metformin. One patient was further transitioned to lifestyle changes only because of hypoglycemia while on metformin and remained euglycemic off medications for at least 1 year before the case report. Both patients had multiple family members with diabetes requiring metformin; however, there are limited genetic data or clinical features documented for the other family members. In addition to research on the currently U.S. Food and Drug Administration–approved diabetes medications, there has been research on gene therapy using lentivirus to transduce IPF1 into heterozygous IPF1 rat hepatocyte cells and targeting Nip3-like protein X (Nix) transcription suppression. This research has had encouraging results of improved glycemic control and abrogated islet β-cell apoptosis in respective studies.

In conclusion, MODY-4 is a rare type of diabetes. Here, we presented a ~30-year overview of the progression and treatment regimen of a patient with MODY-4. Presentation of MODY-4 can include both nonobese and obese patients, with later age of diabetes diagnosis averaging around 35 years old but occasionally up to 50 years old. Treatment is similar to other forms of MODY through lifestyle changes and oral antihyperglycemic drugs based on limited data. It is important to distinguish MODY from other types of diabetes, since management and diabetes progression will differ. Also, because of the atypical presentation of MODY-4, we should consider testing not only patients who are stereotypical of MODY presentation (younger, nonobese, and with no ketosis), but also consider testing patients who are obese, are slightly older than expected, and have a multigenerational vertical family history of diabetes, since this population can often be misdiagnosed as having type 2 diabetes.

COMMENTARY

As the authors of this case correctly pointed out, MODY-4 is a very rare condition. It is always extremely helpful to see the exact mutation (in this case, IPF1 mutation c.784C>A [p.Pro262Thr]) and to compare it with previously published mutations. The family described by Fajans et al.[2] and several individuals with identical mutations in other families all turned out to be cryptically related (undetected mutations).

This patient's glycemia is well controlled with Medtronic 670G insulin pump and yet the patient has developed some chronic complications of diabetes.

Louis H. Philipson, MD, PhD, and Boris Draznin, MD, PhD

REFERENCES

1. Stoffers DA, Ferrer J, Clarke WL, Habener JF. Early-onset type-II diabetes mellitus (MODY4) linked to IPF1. *Nat Genet* 1997;17:138–1392.

2. Fajans SS, Bell GI, Paz VP, et al. Obesity and hyperinsulinemia in a family with pancreatic agenesis and MODY caused by the IPF1 mutation Pro63fsX60. *Transl Res* 2010;156:7–14. doi:10.1016/j.trsl.2010.03.003

3. Deng M, Xiao X, Zhou L, Wang T. First case report of maturity-onset diabetes of the young type 4 pedigree in a Chinese family. *Front Endocrinol* 2019;10:406. doi:10.3389/fendo.2019.00406

4. Yu H, Liu J, Li X, Miao F, Yang Y. Identification of a novel mutation site in maturity onset diabetes of the young in a Chinese family by whole exome sequencing. *Mol Med Rep.* Epub 3 July 2019. doi:10.3892/mmr.2019.10464

Does This Patient Have Type 1 or Type 2 Diabetes?

Zubina Unjom, MD,[1] and Janice L. Gilden, MS, MD[1,2]

A 28-year-old Afro-Caribbean male, with no known prior medical conditions, was recently diagnosed with diabetes after a routine physical examination and blood tests done for pre-employment to prepare for a new, physically demanding job. The initial screening blood glucose level was 465 mg/dL, with an HbA$_{1c}$ of 8.8% (normal 4.0–6.0%). The primary care physician started him on metformin therapy at 1,000 mg twice daily and also placed a referral for dietary consultation. The patient was then referred to the endocrine clinic for further management of diabetes. He denied any symptoms of hyper- or hypoglycemia, infections, emotional or physical stress, or prior knowledge of glucose intolerance and had no family history of diabetes or other autoimmune conditions.

The patient was normotensive with a BMI of 24 kg/m^2, and the remainder of his physical examination was also within normal limits. A funduscopic exam confirmed by an ophthalmologist, and a neurological exam including vibration and monofilament, were without abnormalities. Laboratory results are shown in Table 3.1.

Metformin was discontinued, and the patient was started on basal-bolus insulin therapy. The doses were adjusted to achieve target blood glucose ranges.

It has been recognized that many patients do not fit the classical definitions for the various types of diabetes, as in this patient's case, highlighting the difficulty in distinguishing between type 1 diabetes and type 2 diabetes.

Our patient was a young mascular athletic male with normal body weight and negative GAD65 and islet cell antibodies (ICAs). However, C-peptide level was low with a markedly elevated blood glucose level. C-peptide is often undetectable in patients with type 1 diabetes and is normal to high in type 2 diabetes. Our patient had negative antibodies, thus making it difficult to determine which type of diabetes he might have.

[1]Diabetes/Endocrinology Section, Chicago Medical School, Rosalind Franklin University of Medicine and Science. [2]Captain James A. Lovell Federal Health Care Center, North Chicago, Illinois.

DOI: 10.2337/9781580407663.03

Table 3.1 — Laboratory results

Laboratory Test	Initial Test Results (range)	Repeat Test Results (range)
Fasting blood glucose (mg/dL)	465 (70–90)	383 (70–90)
HbA$_{1c}$ (%)	8.8 (4.0–6.0)	9.3 (4.0–6.0)
Fructosamine (μmol/L)	351 (205–285)	—
Urine ketones	Negative	—
C-peptide (ng/mL)	0.11 (0.81–3.85)	0.07 (0.81–3.85)
Total insulin (mIU/mL)	15 (2.6–24.9)	—
Islet cell antibodies	Negative	—
GAD antibodies	Negative	—
Cholesterol (mg/dL)	79 (0–150)	—
HDL (mg/dL)	34 (>40)	—
Anti-TPO antibody (units/mL)	33.7 (0–60)	—
Anti-Tg antibody (units/mL)	<15 (0–60)	—

Typically, the age of onset for type 1 diabetes is <35 years. In the past, it was presumed that type 2 diabetes would only occur in the adult population, age >35 years. However, in recent years, there has been a change, attributed to the obesity epidemic, with associated increasing incidence of childhood obesity, leading to the development of type 2 diabetes occurring earlier in life.[1]

Type 1 diabetes typically presents with polyuria and polydipsia. Diabetic ketoacidosis is often the initial presentation. Individuals, especially adults with type 1 diabetes, may have other autoimmune diseases, such as celiac disease, Hashimoto's thyroiditis, and vitiligo. This patient did not have any other disorders. The antibodies associated with the development of type 1 diabetes are ICAs, insulin autoantibodies (IAAs), GAD65, zinc transporter 8 (ZnT8), and protein tyrosine phosphatase (IA-2). β-Cell destruction rate can be variable and is often seen to be at an increased rate in children and slower in adults. However, this patient did not have antibodies, nor any other autoimmune disorders.

Another form of diabetes commonly observed in ethnic minorities is latent autoimmune diabetes in adults (LADA). Patients with LADA often present with features of both type 1 and type 2 diabetes. There is often a lower BMI in LADA patients than in patients with type 2 diabetes. In addition, patients with LADA also often have low C-peptide levels. Thus, the following criteria are used for diagnosing LADA: *1)* adult age of onset (>30 years), *2)* presence of any ICAs, and *3)* absence of insulin requirement for at least 6 months.

Table 3.2—Comparison of different characteristics for distinguishing the types of diabetes

	T1D	T2D	LADA
Age (years)	<35	>35	>30
BMI	Normal	Overweight	Normal
C-peptide	Very low	Normal to high	Low
ICAs	Often positive	Negative	Can be positive
GAD antibodies	Often positive	Negative	Can be positive
IA-2	Often positive	Negative	Can be positive
IAAs	Often positive	Negative	Can be positive
HLA link	High	Negative	Low
Time to require insulin	At onset	Can be many years	Within 6 months

A new classification for the types of diabetes has recently been proposed, based on abnormal β-cell function, either due to reduced β-cell mass or a functional decline, as the primary defect leading to hyperglycemia.[2] This classification system focuses on the interaction between genetics, environmental factors, and immune system function.

It is important to take into account the natural history of β-cell mass and functional decline, since this may help to identify the interventions that are required.[3] Thomas et al.[4] suggest that patients diagnosed with diabetes after 30 years of age, who progress to require insulin within the first 3 years of diagnosis, have a higher chance of having type 1 diabetes.

There is also a proposed subclassification of type 1 diabetes. The three stages are stage 1, detection of autoantibodies; stage 2, glucose intolerance; and stage 3, clinically symptomatic. An understanding of these stages may also assist in developing preventive measures and more effective therapies.[5]

This case highlights the difficulty providers may face when trying to establish the correct type of diabetes a particular patient may have and the reasons that patients can often be initially misdiagnosed. It is also common for many patients to be diagnosed with type 2 diabetes, but later discover that they have type 1 diabetes or LADA. The correct diagnosis of type of diabetes has important implications for prescribing the appropriate pharmacological therapy. In the current patient case, metformin therapy had little effect on blood glucose levels, calling into question whether he had type 1 or type 2 diabetes. Based on guidelines of the Immunology of Diabetes Society, this patient did not meet the criteria for LADA. Furthermore, this case also highlights the controversies of the classification system for distinguishing the specific types of diabetes.

COMMENTARY

For the sake of completeness, this interesting case subject should have been evaluated for genetic mutations. Some forms of MODY are de novo mutations, and it is also possible that there is mis-assignment of parentage in some cases without a family history. This case underscores the difficulty providers may face when trying to establish the correct type of diabetes a particular patient may have and the reasons why these patients can often be initially misdiagnosed. It is not uncommon for many patients to be diagnosed with type 2 diabetes but later discover they have type 1 diabetes, LADA, or MODY. Thus, genetic evaluation for the presence of atypical diabetes is almost always in order in such complex and unusual cases.

Louis H. Philipson, MD, PhD, and Boris Draznin, MD, PhD

REFERENCES

1. American Diabetes Association. 2. Classification and diagnosis of diabetes: *Standards of Medical Care in Diabetes—2020. Diabetes Care* 2020;43 (Suppl. 1):S14–S31. https://doi.org/10.2337/dc20-S002.

2. Schwartz SS, Epstein S, Corkey GE, Grant SFA, Gavin JR 3rd, Aguillar RB. The time is right for a new classification system for diabetes: rationale and implications of the β-cell–centric classification schema. *Diabetes Care* 2016;39:179–186

3. Skyler JS, Bakris GL, Bonifacio E, et al. Differentiation of diabetes by pathophysiology, natural history, and prognosis. *Diabetes* 2017;66:241–255

4. Thomas NJ, Lynam AL, Hill AV, et al. Type 1 diabetes defined by severe insulin deficiency occurs after 30 years of age and is commonly treated as type 2 diabetes. *Diabetologia* 2019;62:1167–1172. doi: 10.1007/s00125-019-4863-8. Epub 10 April 2019

5. Insel RA, Dunne JL, Atkinson MA, et al. Staging presymptomatic type 1 diabetes: a scientific statement of JDRF, the Endocrine Society, and the American Diabetes Association. *Diabetes Care* 2015;38:1964–1974

Case 4

Is This an Unusual Type of Diabetes?

Nitish Singh Nandu, MD,[1] Andriy Havrylyan, MD,[1]
Janice L. Gilden, MS, MD,[1,2] and Bushra Osmani, MBBS[3]

A 44-year-old African American female with a history of Graves' hyperthyroidism, now with hypothyroidism after total thyroidectomy, vitiligo, hyperprolactinemia, and orthostatic hypotension due to autonomic neuropathy, presented to the endocrine clinic for reevaluation. She recently noted a new symptom of blurry vision, although she had no other symptoms suggestive of hyper- or hypoglycemia. She also expressed concern about the possibility of developing diabetes, since she had a strong family history of this disorder, with many members suffering chronic complications.

The patient's BMI was 30.3 kg/m² with a body weight of 199 lb. Her physical examination was otherwise unremarkable. Laboratory tests revealed a fasting blood glucose level of 111 mg/dL and HbA$_{1c}$ level of 6.3%. GAD65 antibodies were >30 IU/mL, with a normal C-peptide level of 1.28 ng/mL (normal 0.81–3.85 ng/mL). Continuous glucose monitor testing was performed, revealing normal fasting and preprandial values, but elevations in postprandial blood glucose levels. A diagnosis of type 1 diabetes was made, and she was initially prescribed insulin therapy (detemir 1 unit daily). This dose was up-titrated gradually to 6 units daily, based on blood glucose and HbA$_{1c}$ levels ranging from 6.0 to 6.4%. Because of fears of developing chronic complications, the patient made a drastic change in her diet and increased her physical activity over the next several years. She lost 86 lb, ultimately weighing 115 lb, with a BMI of 17.5 kg/m². She was subsequently diagnosed with an eating disorder and was enrolled in an adult eating disorder treatment program.

The patient then developed episodes of hypoglycemia, particularly on days that she exercised. Although the insulin doses were decreased, she had a fall, presumably due to hypoglycemia, and suffered a jaw fracture, which further aggravated her eating disorder. Despite the reduction in her insulin dosage, she continued to have hypoglycemic episodes with blood glucose levels in the 40s, and insulin therapy was eventually discontinued. Her HbA$_{1c}$ decreased to 4.3%. She continued to remain off insulin therapy over

[1]Diabetes/Endocrinology Section, Chicago Medical School at Rosalind Franklin University of Medicine and Science. [2]Captain James A. Lovell Federal Health Care Center, North Chicago, Illinois. [3]Community Physicians at Froedtert and the Medical College of Wisconsin at Milwaukee, Milwaukee, Wisconsin.

 DOI: 10.2337/9781580407663.04

Table 4.1 — GAD65 trends

Time Level	GAD65 (IU/mL)
At the time of diagnosis	>30
2-Month follow-up	>30
2-Year follow-up	>30
5-Year follow-up	>250
7-Year follow-up	>250

the next 3 years. However, repeat laboratory tests showed a persistent elevation in GAD65 antibodies (Table 4.1) with normal C-peptide levels. Currently, the patient continues to follow a low-carbohydrate diet and reports no further hypoglycemic episodes and has remained off insulin therapy for over 4 years (Table 4.2).

Diabetes, a chronic condition of impaired blood glucose metabolism, results from an impairment in insulin secretion, an abnormal insulin sensitivity, and/or insulin resistance and is broadly classified into four main categories (Table 4.3).[1]

Latent autoimmune diabetes in adults (LADA), or autoimmune (AI) diabetes, is a subtype of type 1 diabetes, defined by three features: onset in adults, the presence of diabetes-associated autoantibodies, and a delay in the need for insulin from the time of diagnosis to management of hyperglycemia.[2] Despite the presence of islet antibodies, the progression of autoimmune β-cell failure is slow in LADA. LADA exhibits characteristics of both type 1 and type 2 diabetes and is sometimes referred to as type 1.5 diabetes.[3] About 5–15% of adults diagnosed with diabetes are often misdiagnosed with type 2 diabetes, but have type 1 diabetes or LADA.[4] The presence of specific autoantibodies directed against pancreatic β-cells helps differentiate LADA from type 2 diabetes, with the most sensitive antibody marker being GAD65 autoantibodies. Other

Table 4.2 — Patient characteristics

	At time of diagnosis	2-Year follow-up	5-Year follow-up	7-Year follow-up
Body weight (lb)	190	162	126	118.6
BMI (kg/m²)	28.04	30.32	21.33	17.55
HbA$_{1c}$ (%)	6.30	6.10	6.00	6.60

Table 4.3—Classification of types of diabetes

Type 1 Diabetes	Type 2 Diabetes	Gestational Diabetes	Diabetes from Secondary Causes
- From Autoimmune β-cell destruction, leading to insulin deficiency - From latent auto-immune diabetes in adults (LADA)	From progressive loss of adequate β-cell insulin secretion in the background of insulin resistance	Commonly manifests in second or third trimester of pregnancy in women without any previous diagnosis; has the potential to progress to overt diabetes	- Monogenic diabetes syndromes (neonatal diabetes, maturity-onset diabetes of the young) - Disease of the exocrine pancreas (cystic fibrosis, pancreatitis) or pancreatectomy - Drug-induced causes (from chronic gluco corticoid therapy, HIV/AIDS, or after organ transplant)

antibodies such as cytoplasmic islet cell antibodies (ICAs), insulin autoantibodies (IAAs), protein tyrosine phosphatase IA-2 antibodies, and islet-specific zinc transporter 8 (ZnT8) autoantibodies are also seen.

There is great variability in how AI diabetes presents in a clinical setting, ranging from fasting hyperglycemia to overt diabetic ketoacidosis on initial presentation. Because the disease progression in LADA occurs at a slower pace than in classic type 1 diabetes, therapy should be aimed at delaying β-cell failure. Studies are ongoing to determine if early initiation of insulin or the use of immunomodulatory therapy can prevent disease progression.

Thus, properly identifying the specific type of diabetes for the patient determines the most appropriate treatment regimen. However, sometimes a patient cannot be clearly classified. For example, a patient with LADA may be misdiagnosed and treated with therapies commonly used for type 2 diabetes, which might further worsen the autoimmune process and accelerate β-cell loss. This misdiagnosis leads to faster progression and the need for insulin therapy.[5] Therefore, physicians and other providers should be cautious to keep the various etiologies in mind when treating diabetes. This case highlights the difficulty often encountered in determining the correct type of diabetes, which has important implications not only for therapeutic and psychosocial interventions, but also for the expectations for disease progression and the risk for chronic complications.

COMMENTARY

This case is an interesting occurrence of diabetes with ketosis in a setting of poly-autoimmunity and anti-GAD positivity. A remarkable feature of this study is that, over time, the patient was able to be titrated off of insulin over years with persistent anti-GAD antibodies of high titer. Close follow-up with attention to recurrent hyperglycemia is clearly needed. This case report is a good discussion of variability in LADA and overlap with other forms of diabetes.

Louis H. Philipson, MD, PhD, and Boris Draznin, MD, PhD

REFERENCES

1. American Diabetes Association. 2. Classification and diagnosis of diabetes: *Standards of Medical Care in Diabetes—2020*. *Diabetes Care* 2020;43(Suppl. 1): S14–S31. doi:10.2337/dc20-S002

2. Leslie RDG, Williams R, Pozzilli P. Clinical review: type 1 diabetes and latent autoimmune diabetes in adults: one end of the rainbow. *J Clin Endocrinol Metab* 2006;91:1654–1659. doi:10.1210/jc.2005-1623

3. Basile KJ, Guy VC, Schwartz S, Grant SFA. Overlap of genetic susceptibility to type 1 diabetes, type 2 diabetes, and latent autoimmune diabetes in adults. *Curr Diab Rep* 2014;14:550. doi:10.1007/s11892-014-0550-9

4. Stenström G, Gottsäter A, Bakhtadze E, Berger B, Sundkvist G. Latent auto-immune diabetes in adults. *Diabetes* 2005;54(Suppl. 2):S68–S72. doi:10.2337/diabetes.54.suppl_2.S68

5. Buzzetti R, Zampetti S, Maddaloni E. Adult-onset autoimmune diabetes: current knowledge and implications for management. *Nat Rev Endocrinol* 2017;13:674–686. doi:10.1038/nrendo.2017.99

Challenges in the Management of Pancreatogenic (Type 3c) Diabetes

Katrina Han, MD,[1] and Janet B. McGill, MD[1]

A 33-year-old female with a history of hereditary pancreatitis and type 3c diabetes was admitted to the hospital with abdominal pain and nausea. The endocrine service was consulted for inpatient management of diabetes.

She experienced her first episode of pancreatitis at the age of 5 and was soon after diagnosed with hereditary pancreatitis. On genetic testing, she was found to have an R122H PRSS1 (protease serine 1) variant, which is an activating mutation in trypsinogen and the most common variant in patients with autosomal-dominant hereditary pancreatitis. She underwent a partial pancreatectomy and jejunostomy at age 14 but continued to have chronic abdominal pain and recurrent pancreatitis episodes, requiring chronic opioids for pain management. Persistent abdominal pain impeded her ability to maintain consistent follow-up. This sporadic treatment contributed to inadequate compliance with her diabetes regimen. Issues with insurance and medication cost led to inconsistent treatment with oral pancreatic enzyme replacement therapy.

Her history was also notable for pregnancy at age 31, complicated by poorly controlled diabetes, pancreatitis, and preterm labor with non-reassuring fetal status, requiring emergent cesarean section with partial sacral agenesis of the fetus.

On admission, she endorsed a 3-day history of worsening abdominal pain, postprandial nausea, and inability to tolerate oral intake, similar to her prior episodes of acute on chronic pancreatitis. She also noted intermittent diarrhea/steatorrhea. She reported compliance with a low-fat diet before the onset of her symptoms. Exam was notable for abdominal tenderness. She weighed 130.3 lb (BMI 27.1 kg/m²). Laboratory studies were notable for an elevated HbA$_{1c}$ of 15.1% (normal <5.7%) and low lipase level of <3 units/L (normal range 10–99 units/L). Vitamin levels were checked and showed vitamin A 17.1 µg/dL (normal range 32.5–78.0 µg/dL), 25-hydroxyvitamin D 14 ng/mL (normal range 30–80 ng/mL), vitamin E 1.9 mg/L (normal range 5.5–17.0 mg/L), and vitamin K <0.03 ng/mL (normal range

[1]Division of Endocrinology, Metabolism, and Lipid Research, Washington University School of Medicine, St. Louis, Missouri.

 DOI: 10.2337/9781580407663.05

0.10–2.20 ng/mL). A computed tomography scan of the abdomen and pelvis demonstrated an atrophic remnant pancreas with calcifications, consistent with chronic pancreatitis.

The patient's insulin doses were adjusted to maintain blood glucose levels within the target range of 140–180 mg/dL, with final doses of 10 units insulin glargine daily and 4 units insulin lispro three times daily with meals. Oral pancreatic enzyme replacement therapy with 24,000 units pancrelipase (Creon) three times daily with meals was initiated with a reduction in steatorrhea. She was also started on 8,000 units vitamin A daily, 1,000 units vitamin E daily, 50,000 units ergocalciferol (vitamin D2) weekly, and 5 mg phytonadione (vitamin K) weekly. Education was provided on recommended dietary intake, including oral nutritional supplements, and the importance of taking pancreatic enzymes with meals and snacks.

Patients who have developed insulin-deficient diabetes secondary to chronic pancreatitis are at high risk of having coexisting pancreatic exocrine insufficiency. To optimize diabetes treatment in patients with chronic pancreatitis and pancreatic exocrine insufficiency, tailored medical nutrition therapy, use of pancreatic enzyme replacement, and vitamin supplements to treat micronutrient deficiencies may all be required. The main goals of medical nutrition therapy are to prevent or treat malnutrition, reduce fat malabsorption, and limit meal-induced hyperglycemia.[1]

Initiation of oral pancreatic enzyme replacement therapy when pancreatic exocrine insufficiency is identified is crucial to achieving these goals. Pancreatic enzyme replacement improves fat absorption, which helps to control the symptoms of steatorrhea and diminish the loss of fat-soluble vitamins A, D, E, and K. It also restores the secretion of intestine-derived incretin hormones, including glucagon-like peptide-1. This result leads to improved glucose-dependent insulin secretion, which may help to reduce postprandial hyperglycemia in patients with residual functioning β-cells.[2,3] Furthermore, some studies have shown that pancreatic enzyme replacement may reduce abdominal pain[4]; however, studies are not consistent regarding pain reduction. Proposed mechanisms include feedback inhibition of pancreatic secretion; improved fat digestion, which reduces symptoms associated with malabsorption; and alteration of nutrition-microbiome interactions.

Deficiencies in other micronutrients, including vitamin B12, zinc, calcium, magnesium, thiamine, and folic acid, have also been reported and are important to address in patients with chronic pancreatitis.[5] Despite the known importance of nutrition, no formal guidelines exist for the optimal diet and nutritional supplement regimen for patients with type 3c diabetes. Some groups recommend frequent small meals (four to eight times a day) and daily fat intake of <30 g per day with elimination of saturated fats. Medium-chain fatty acids, such as 1–2 tablespoons of palm kernel oil per day, can be added to assist with nutrient absorption and to reduce fatty acid deficiencies, since medium-chain fatty acids are absorbed directly across the small bowel into the portal vein and do not rely on the presence of lipase, co-lipase, or bile salts. A low-fiber diet has also been recommended, since dietary fiber can absorb and prevent the action of pancreatic enzymes.[5]

Of note, patients with type 3c diabetes are at higher risk for hypoglycemia because of decreased muscle mass and deficient counter-regulatory glucagon secretion. Thus, insulin doses must be carefully titrated, and the administration of short-acting insulin agents must be appropriately timed before meal ingestion to prevent hypoglycemic events.

In conclusion, type 3c diabetes remains an underrecognized, often-misclassified, and clinically challenging condition that tends to be suboptimally managed. These patients have complex nutritional needs and require close monitoring to ensure an adequate and balanced intake of micro- and macronutrients. Oral pancreatic enzyme replacement therapy remains a cornerstone of treatment and should be initiated at the time of diagnosis of pancreatic exocrine deficiency to help prevent malnutrition and to improve glycemic control. Coordinated treatment with medical nutrition therapy and appropriate timing of insulin administration are essential to improving clinical outcomes for patients with type 3c diabetes.

COMMENTARY

This study is an interesting and rare case of hereditary pancreatitis with the PRSS1 mutation. Usually, elevated levels of trypsin in the pancreas result in significant damage to pancreatic tissue. There is an increased risk for pancreatic cancer in patients with hereditary pancreatitis.

Hereditary pancreatitis is a chronic, progressive disease and, unfortunately, there is no cure. Recently, total pancreatectomy with islet autotransplantation has emerged as an option for treatment of patients with debilitating pain. Short of this option, patients with type 3c diabetes are treated with insulin, and special attention is needed to avoid hypoglycemia, as is well presented in this case.

Louis H. Philipson, MD, PhD, and Boris Draznin, MD, PhD

REFERENCES

1. Rickels MR, Bellin M, Toledo FG, et al. Detection, evaluation and treatment of diabetes mellitus in chronic pancreatitis: recommendations from Pancreas Fest 2012. *Pancreatology* 2013;13:336–342

2. Ebert R, Creutzfeldt W. Reversal of impaired GIP and insulin secretion in patients with pancreatogenic steatorrhea following enzyme substitution. *Diabetologia* 1980;19:198–204

3. Knop FK, Vilsboll T, Larsen S, et al. Increased postprandial responses of GLP-1 and GIP in patients with chronic pancreatitis and steatorrhea following pancreatic enzyme substitution. *Am J Physiol Endocrinol Metab* 2007;292:E324–E330

4. Larvin M, McMahon MJ, Thomas WEG, Puntis MCA. Creon (enteric coated pancreatic microspheres) for the treatment of pain in chronic pancreatitis: a double blind randomized placebo controlled crossover study. *Gastroenterology* 1991;100:A283

5. Duggan SN, Ewald N, Kelleher L, et al. The nutritional management of type 3c (pancreatogenic) diabetes in chronic pancreatitis. *Eur J Clin Nutr* 2017;71:3–8

Case 6

New-Onset Diabetes as a Symptom of Pancreatic Adenocarcinoma

Emily Gammoh, MD,[1] and Jagdeesh Ullal, MD[1]

The case subject was a 59-year-old male with no past medical history who was admitted with diabetic ketoacidosis. He gave a history of unintentional weight loss of 20 lb over 3 months, which was associated with fatigue and weakness. A couple of weeks before presentation, he started to develop polyuria and polydipsia. His family history included type 2 diabetes on his mother's side of the family. He also had a 10-pack-year history of smoking but quit 2–3 years prior. On examination, the patient was a thin male (BMI 22 kg/m^2) with stable vital signs and mild epigastric tenderness, but exam was otherwise unremarkable. Laboratory findings were significant for a bicarbonate level of 14 mEq/L, blood glucose of 312 mg/dL, acetone in the serum, and anion gap of 17 mEq/L, suggestive of ketoacidosis. HbA$_{1c}$ was 13.5%. He was treated with intravenous fluids and an insulin drip, which was later transitioned to basal-bolus insulin. Along with recommending type 1 diabetes antibody testing, our team recommended pancreatic imaging considering his age, weight loss, and newly diagnosed diabetes. A computed tomography (CT) scan of the abdomen and pelvis revealed a lobulated 3.6 × 3.3 × 2.8 cm mixed-density/hypo-enhancing mass in the distal pancreatic tail. Endoscopic ultrasound (EUS)-guided biopsy revealed ductal type pancreatic adenocarcinoma. The patient's CA 19-9 (cancer antigen 19-9) level was 10,398.3 units/mL. Two weeks after the initial CT, repeat imaging revealed multiple hypodense lesions in the liver, not previously seen. Magnetic resonance imaging revealed intracranial metastasis in the clivus, consistent with a diagnosis of stage IV pancreatic adenocarcinoma. Over the next 3 weeks, CA 19-9 increased further to >20,000 units/mL. The patient maintained tight glucose control as an outpatient, and his HbA$_{1c}$ improved to 6.7% 5 months later. The patient did not have symptoms of exocrine dysfunction such as diarrhea or steatorrhea and did not need initiation of pancreatic enzymes. The pancreatic adenocarcinoma was initially treated with FOLFIRINOX (5-fluorouracil, leucovorin, irinotecan, and oxaliplatin) chemotherapy, but his scans showed further progression in less than 3 months, indicating aggressive cancer. He was switched to gemcitabine

[1]University of Pittsburgh School of Medicine, University of Pittsburgh Medical Center, Center for Diabetes and Endocrinology, Pittsburgh, Pennsylvania.

 DOI: 10.2337/9781580407663.06

and abraxane. He also received radiation therapy for clival metastasis. His current goal of therapy is to maximize quality of life given the incurable nature of his disease.

The relationship between diabetes and pancreatic adenocarcinoma is complex and has yet to be fully understood. Diabetes has long been recognized as a risk factor for pancreatic cancer, but more recent studies have shown a stronger correlation, with the development of diabetes preceding the diagnosis of pancreatic cancer. This result is hypothesized to occur not only secondary to glandular destruction, but also to increased insulin resistance, β-cell dysfunction caused by toxic secretory products of the cancer cells, and immunopathogenesis.[1] A more recent study showed that the relative risk of being diagnosed with pancreatic cancer within 1 year of a diabetes diagnosis was 6.91 (95% CI 5.76–8.30), whereas the relative risk among patients with longstanding diabetes was 1.96 (95% CI 1.62–2.38), which points to the likelihood that new-onset diabetes may be a harbinger of underlying pancreatic cancer.[2]

Pancreatic adenocarcinoma is a devastating diagnosis with a 5-year survival rate of <5%.[3] There is mounting evidence that new-onset diabetes may be an early sign of an underlying pancreatic cancer, with the diagnosis of diabetes preceding the cancer diagnosis by an average of 10 months.[3] Pannala et al.[4] also found that 50% of patients with stage I and II pancreatic cancer have diabetes. Currently, the U.S. Preventive Services Task Force does not recommend the screening of asymptomatic patients, including those with new-onset diabetes, older age, smoking history, obesity, etc. Although around 30–50% of patients with pancreatic cancer have concurrent diabetes, <1% of patients with new-onset diabetes have pancreatic cancer, making testing not cost-effective in this population.[4] There is no reliable biomarker available for the screening of pancreatic cancer. Hence, screening would require radiologic testing such as contrast-enhanced CT scans or EUS. Sharma et al.[5] at the Mayo Clinic recently developed the Enriching New-Onset Diabetes for Pancreatic Cancer (END-PAC) model based on three previously noted features that distinguished type 2 diabetes from pancreatic cancer–associated diabetes: first, weight gain versus weight loss; second, slow progression from normal fasting glucose to type 2 diabetes (occurring over around 8 years) (whereas pancreatic cancer–associated diabetes is more rapidly progressive); and, third, patients with type 2 diabetes are typically younger than patients with pancreatic cancer–associated diabetes." This model provides some reassurance that patients with a score <0 may not likely need to be considered for screening.[5] However, there are limitations to the model: it uses historical blood glucose and weight recorded 1 year before diagnosis, which may not be easily available. An END-PAC score of ≥3 had a sensitivity of 78% and specificity of 82%; these results enriched the pancreatic cancer prevalence of 0.82% in the population-based cohort to 3.6%. In the patients with an END-PAC score of 1–2, 0.54% developed pancreatic cancer within 3 years, whereas the patients with a score of ≤0 did not develop pancreatic cancer. Further development of this screening model is needed to select appropriate patients for screening, with higher probability of early diagnosis and improved survival while avoiding overuse of medical procedures.

While diabetes associated with pancreatic cancer is generally considered a form of type 3c diabetes, or pancreatogenic diabetes, the strong association between new-onset diabetes and a deadly form of cancer deserves more scrutiny and guidelines to address screening. While type 3c diabetes is associated with fibrosis and loss of islet mass, islet function is generally preserved until a large part of exocrine function is reduced. As demonstrated in our patient, diabetes developed before the development of major pancreatic exocrine function loss, which alludes to possible humoral mechanisms of islet damage in conjunction with previously understood mechanisms of type 3c diabetes etiology. Outcomes of the Consortium for the Study of Chronic Pancreatitis, Diabetes and Pancreatic Cancer (CPDPC) will provide direction in the complex association of new-onset diabetes and pancreatic cancer.[1]

COMMENTARY

Among the several interesting points of this case, one is probably the most important. Clearly, type 1 diabetes can manifest at any age and present itself as ketoacidosis. This, however, should not detract an astute clinician from examining the potential causes of this initial presentation. In this case, a timely CT scan was instrumental in uncovering the patient's pancreatic adenocarcinoma.

Boris Draznin, MD, PhD

REFERENCES

1. Serrano J, Andersen DK, Forsmark CE, et al. Consortium for the Study of Chronic Pancreatitis, Diabetes, and Pancreatic Cancer: from concept to reality. *Pancreas* 2018;47:1208–1212

2. Huang BZ, Pandol SJ, Jeon CY, et al. New-onset diabetes, longitudinal trends in metabolic markers, and risk of pancreatic cancer in a heterogeneous population. *Clin Gastroenterol Hepatol* 2020;18:1812–1821

3. Pelaez-Luna M, Takahashi N, Fletcher JG, Chari ST. Resectability of presymptomatic pancreatic cancer and its relationship to onset of diabetes: a retrospective review of CT scans and fasting glucose values prior to diagnosis. *Am J Gastroenterol* 2007;102:2157–2163

4. Pannala R, Leirness JB, Bamlet WR, Basu A, Petersen GM, Chari ST. Prevalence and clinical profile of pancreatic cancer-associated diabetes mellitus. *Gastroenterology* 2008;134:981–987

5. Sharma A, Kandlakunta H, Nagpal SJS, et al. Model to determine risk of pancreatic cancer in patients with new-onset diabetes. *Gastroenterology* 2018;155:730–739.e3

Case 7

Sweet's Syndrome in a Patient With Diabetes

Nitish Singh Nandu, MD,[1] Sabah Patel, MD,[2] and Janice L. Gilden, MS, MD[1,2]

A 66-year-old male patient with type 2 diabetes, peripheral neuropathy, orthostatic hypotension due to autonomic neuropathy, hyperlipidemia, and chronic obstructive pulmonary disease was evaluated by endocrinology for continuing diabetes management. His complaints were dizziness with frequent falls and decreased sensation in his lower extremities.

He had diabetes for the past 11 years, with blood glucose values ranging from 150–490 mg/dL and HbA$_{1c}$ of 8.4–14.1%. He reported poor compliance with diet and medications. Five years previously, he was diagnosed with peripheral neuropathy and orthostatic hypotension due to autonomic dysfunction. These symptoms were presumed to be as a result of his poorly controlled diabetes. Although he smoked cigarettes, he had no other significant contributory social or family history.

On physical examination, he had a rash on the upper extremities. He attributed the rash to prolonged sun exposure and reported the same rash on other various areas of his body occurring over the past 4 years. His current medication regimen included saxagliptin, insulin detemir, midodrine, and pregabalin. On physical examination, he was afebrile and had orthostatic hypotension with a decrease in blood pressure from 104/50 to 69/46 mmHg and increase in heart rate from 72 to 118 beats/min. There was also diminished pinprick and vibration sensation in his lower extremities. The rash on his dorsal hands and forearms appeared lichenified and indurated with annular plaques, with hemorrhagic crusting and central ulcerations (Laboratory data are summarized in Figure 7.1).

Therefore, he was referred to dermatology for a skin biopsy, which showed dense band-like infiltrates located in the papillary and upper reticular dermis, characteristic of Sweet's syndrome (Figure 7.2). An investigation for occult malignancies was negative, and the patient was not taking any of the medications known to cause Sweet's syndrome. Treatment with systemic corticosteroids was deferred because of the labile and poorly controlled blood glucose levels. Therefore, he was initially started on topical triamcinolone therapy. However, because of a poor response to treatment

[1]Diabetes/Endocrinology Section, Chicago Medical School at Rosalind Franklin University of Medicine and Science. [2]Captain James A. Lovell Federal Health Care Center, North Chicago, Illinois.

DOI: 10.2337/9781580407663.07

Table 7.1—Laboratory data

		Reference
Glucose (mg/dL)	305	70–99
HbA$_{1c}$ (%)	7.4	4.0–6.0
Blood urea nitrogen (mg/dL)	23	7–21
Creatinine (mg/dL)	1.040	0.67–1.17
Sodium (mmol/L)	132	136–145
Potassium (mmol/L)	4.7	3.5–4.7
Chloride (mmol/L)	101	98–107
CO_2 (mmol/L)	24	21–32
Anion gap (mmol/L)	12	8–20
Calcium (mg/dL)	9.6	8.5–10.1
AST (units/L)	6	10–37
ALT (units/L)	19	10–65
Alkaline phosphatase (units/L)	245	45–117
Total bilirubin (mg/dL)	0.6	0.2–1.0
Gamma-GTP (units/L)	10	15–85
Cholesterol (mg/dL)	235	0–200
Triglycerides (mg/dL)	179	0–150
HDL cholesterol (mg/dL)	51	≥40
LDL cholesterol (mg/dL)	148	0–100
Thyroid-stimulating hormone (μIU/mL)	2.38	0.358–3.74
Free T4 (ng/dL)	1.08	0.76–1.46
B-HCG (mIU/mL)	<2	<5
ANA screen	Positive	
Anti-SSA (EU)	1.70	0–19
Anti-SSB (EU)	0.37	0–19
Anti-dsDNA antibody (IU)	4.73	0–24
Cardiolipin panel	Negative	
Rheumatoid factor (IU/mL)	<10	0–15
P-ANCA	0.46	<0.90
C-ANCA	0.14	≤0.90
Kappa light chains (mg/dL)	230	176–443
Lambda LC (mg/dL)	118	176–443

Table 7.1—*continued*

BCR-ABL	Negative	
Beta 2 microglobulin	Negative	
Hepatitis B core antibody	Nonreactive	
Hepatitis B surface antigen	Nonreactive	
HIV1/2	Nonreactive	
White blood cells (K/μL)	10.5	4.0–11.0
Red blood cells (M/μL)	4.41	4.2–5.70
HGB (g/dL)	13.5	3.0–17.0
HCT (%)	40.8	
MCV (fL)	92.5	82.0–99.0
MCH (pg)	30.6	27.0–34.0
MCHC (g/dL)	33.1	31–37
RDW (%)	14.0	0–15.0
PLT (K/μL)	187	130–400
MPV (fL)	11.5	8.0–12.0
Neutrophils (%)	61.3	40–80
Lymphocytes (%)	28.6	15–45
Monocytes (%)	7.5	2–12
Eosinophils (%)	2.2	0–6
Basophils (%)	0.4	0-2

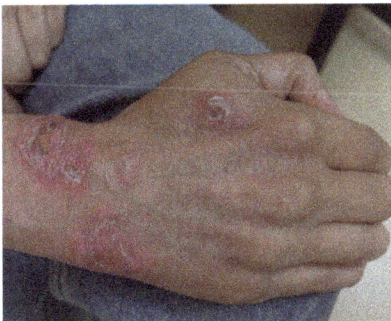

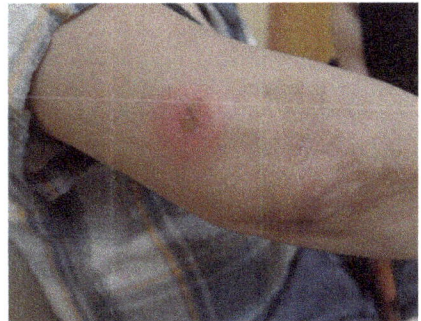

Figure 7.1—The patient's skin lesions as a result of Sweet's syndrome.

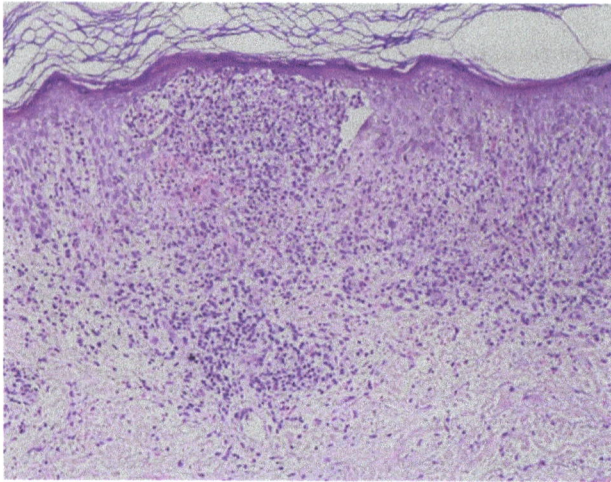

Figure 7.2—A typical histopathology slide of Sweet's syndrome.

and frequent exacerbations, he was switched to topical dapsone, with recommendations to avoid prolonged sun exposure.

Sweet's syndrome, or acute febrile neutrophilic dermatosis, is a rare inflammatory disorder characterized by the abrupt onset of painful erythematous plaques, papules, or nodules of the skin. It is associated with a wide range of disorders that have been grouped into three categories (Table 7.2).[1]

1. Classic Sweet's syndrome: associated with infections, inflammatory disorders, and pregnancy
2. Malignancy-associated Sweet's syndrome: most often with hematologic malignancies
3. Drug-induced Sweet's syndrome

The pathogenesis of Sweet's syndrome remains unclear, although the association with infection, autoimmune diseases, neoplasms, and drugs suggests a hypersensitivity reaction, mediated by cytokines, followed by infiltration of neutrophils likely activated by interleukin-1.[2] It has been theorized that photosensitivity may play a role in the pathogenesis by an unknown mechanism, since Sweet's syndrome was experimentally induced by photo testing.[3] The incidence of Sweet's syndrome may also be underreported, since most patients, like ours, presume it to be a rash or a sunburn. Neurologic manifestations of Sweet's syndrome are rare, with the most common complications being meningitis and encephalitis. Peripheral neuropathy has also been documented in extremely rare scenarios and has been noted to be permanent, despite treatment with corticosteroids.[4] It is difficult to distinguish peripheral neuropathy caused by Sweet's syndrome from that with diabetes. There are also case

Table 7.2—Etiologies of Sweet's syndrome and summary of known causes

Classic Sweet's syndrome	Malignancy-associated Sweet's syndrome	Drug-induced Sweet's syndrome

Infections: Develop 1–3 weeks after the infection
- Upper respiratory tract infections; gastrointestinal infections
- Others
  • HIV
  • Tuberculosis
  • Chlamydia
  • Viral hepatitis
 	
Inflammatory bowel disease
- Crohn's disease
- Ulcerative colitis
 	
Pregnancy
 	
Autoimmune conditions
- Bechet syndrome
- Relapsing polychondritis
- Rheumatoid arthritis
- Sarcoidosis
- Autoimmune thyroid disease
 	
Connective tissue disorders
- Systemic lupus erythematosus
- Dermatomyositis
	Carcinomas of the
	- Genitourinary tract
	- Breast
	- Gastrointestinal tract
	
	Hematologic malignancies
		- Antithyroid hormone synthesis drugs: propylthiouracil
		- Antimicrobials: minocycline, nitrofurantoin, norfloxacin, ofloxacin, quinupristin/dalfopristin, trimethoprim-sulfamethoxazole, abacavir
		- Antihypertensives: hydralazine
		- Antineoplastics: bortezomib, imatinib, ipilimumab, lenalidomide, topotecan, vemurafenib
		- Antipsychotics
		- Clozapine
		- Colony-stimulating factors
		- Granulocyte-colony–stimulating factor, granulocyte-macrophage-colony–stimulating factor, pegfilgrastim
		- Immunosuppressants
		- Azathioprine
		- Nonsteroidal antiinflammatory agents
		- Celecoxib, diclofenac
		- Retinoids
		- All-trans retinoic acid, 13-cis-retinoic acid

reports in the literature of diabetes associated with Sweet's syndrome.[5] It is possible that the neuropathy and autonomic dysfunction noted in our patient was likely due to the combination of Sweet's syndrome and diabetes. Diabetes is a pro-inflammatory state, which can also be a trigger for Sweet's syndrome. However, research documenting a clear causative correlation is lacking. Diabetes also poses an important therapeutic challenge, since systemic corticosteroids are the first-line therapy for Sweet's syndrome, due to increased insulin resistance, which can result in higher blood glucose levels. Thus, their use in patients can lead to worsening glycemic control. Alternative treatments include triamcinolone, indomethacin, clofazimine, cyclosporine, dapsone doxycycline, and pentoxifylline.[1] Further research is essential to better understand the implications of diabetes as a trigger for Sweet's syndrome.

COMMENTARY

Sweet's syndrome is an uncommon disease. It is an inflammatory skin condition characterized by sudden onset of painful rash on the upper and lower extremities, trunk, neck, and face and is accompanied by fever. Histologically, Sweet's syndrome represents neutrophilic dermatosis, and, clinically, it is frequently referred to as acute febrile neutrophilic dermatosis. Corticosteroids are the mainstay of treatment of Sweet's syndrome, which may resolve and recur periodically despite therapy. Treatment with corticosteroids obviously introduces another challenge to diabetes management.

While a description of skin disorders is beyond the scope of this book, we wish to remind our readers that, recently, bullous pemphigoid was described in association with administration of dipeptidyl peptidase-4 inhibitors. Also, necrotizing fasciitis of the perineum on and around genitals was described in association with administration of sodium–glucose cotransporter 2 (SGLT2) inhibitors (Fournier's gangrene).

Louis H. Philipson, MD, PhD, and Boris Draznin, MD, PhD

REFERENCES

1. Cohen PR. Sweet's syndrome: a comprehensive review of an acute febrile neutrophilic dermatosis. *Orphanet J Rare Dis* 2007;2:34. doi:10.1186/1750-1172-2-34

2. Villarreal-Villarreal CD, Ocampo-Candiani J, Villarreal-Martínez A. Sweet syndrome: a review and update. *Actas Dermosifiliogr* 2016;107:369–378. doi: 10.1016/j.ad.2015.12.001

3. Meyer V, Schneider SW, Bonsmann G, Beissert S. Experimentally confirmed induction of Sweet's syndrome by phototesting. *Acta Derm Venereol* 2011;91:720–721. doi: 10.2340/00015555-1139

4. Cala CM, Kole L, Sami N. Bilateral sensorineural hearing loss and polyneuropathy in a patient with Sweet's syndrome. *Case Rep Otolaryngol* 2015;2015:751538. doi: 10.1155/2015/751538

5. Hibiya K, Miyagi K, Tamaose M, et al. Do infections with disseminated Mycobacterium Avium complex pecede sweet's syndrome? A case report and literature review. *Int J Mycobacteriol* 2017;6;336–343. doi: 10.4103/ijmy.ijmy-172-17

This research was supported, in part, by the Captain James A. Lovell Health Care Center.

Case 8:
Wolcott-Rallison Syndrome

MEHMET N. ÖZBEK, MD,[1] AND EDA CENGIZ, MD, MHS, FAAP[2,3]

A 28-month-old girl with a history of type 1 diabetes presented to the emergency room with fever and vomiting. She was diagnosed with type 1 diabetes at 2 months of age and had been being administered multiple daily injections of insulin. Past history was otherwise unremarkable. Family history was unknown, including history of consanguinity. Her vital signs revealed a temperature of 102.2°F, heart rate of 140 beats/min, and respiratory rate of 32/min. Her height was 2.4 ft (–4.54 standard deviation score [SDS]) and weight was 17.2 lb (–3.58 SDS). Physical examination was significant for decreased skin turgor, hyperemic pharynx, and hepatosplenomegaly (3 cm below the right costal margin). Laboratory tests showed blood glucose of 347 mg/dL, serum creatinine of 0.45 mg/dL, ALT of 878 units/L, AST of 2,136 units/L, total bilirubin of 0.45 mg/dL, direct bilirubin of 0.11 mg/dL, hemoglobin of 9.4 g/dL, platelet count of 402.000/mm[3], white blood cell count of 5.500/mm, absolute neutrophil count (ANC) of 890, and C-reactive protein (CRP) of 101.4 mg/L. Blood gas was within normal limits with a normal pH. Intravenous fluid hydration, wide spectrum antibiotic treatment, and insulin treatment were initiated. Blood glucose level came down to 169 mg/dL after hydration and insulin treatment. On the second day of admission, ANC decreased to 127/mm[3]; therefore, subcutaneous granulocyte colony-stimulating factor (G-CSF) treatment was initiated. On the third day of G-CSF treatment, ANC level normalized, and ALT, AST, and CRP declined to 115 units/L, 55 units/L, and 10.1 mg/dL, respectively.

Genetic testing was ordered during admission given the neonatal onset of T1D and showed a homozygous (c.1884-1G>c) mutation in the EIF2AK3 gene, resulting in abnormal aberrant splicing in the acceptor domain of the 11th intron. Review of the patient's medical records revealed history of transient elevation of liver enzymes (ALT 416 units/L, AST 960 units/L) at diabetes onset. Diabetes autoimmune panel results were not available.

[1]Gazi Yasargil Training and Research Hospital Clinics of Pediatric Endocrinology, Diyarbakır, Turkey. [2]Division of Pediatric Endocrinology and Diabetes, Yale School of Medicine, New Haven, Connecticut. [3]Visiting Professor, Bahcesehir University, Istanbul, Turkey.

DOI: 10.2337/9781580407663.08

The patient was seen at the outpatient clinic at 5.5 years of age with a chief complaint of back pain without history of trauma. She had marked growth retardation (height 2.7 ft [-7.68 SDS], mid-parental height 5.2 ft [-0.82 SDS], and weight 27.1 lb [-4.45 SDS]) and an HbA_{1c} of 11.8%, indicative of suboptimal glycemic control. Thyroid function test results showed an elevated thyroid-stimulating hormone level (10.8 vIU/mL), a free T4 at the lower limit of normal (0.98 ng/dL), and negative anti-thyroglobulin and anti-TPO antibodies. Na-L-thyroxine supplementation was started for treatment of hypothyroidism. X-rays revealed acetabular flattening and irregular femoral head epiphyses without any fracture. Dual-energy X-ray absorptiometry showed decreased bone mineral density (Z score -3.9) in the lumbar vertebrae. Pamidronate treatment was started (1 mg/kg every 3 months) for osteoporosis.

The patient was admitted multiple times during the following years with elevated liver enzymes (ALT up to 2,659 units/L and AST up to 4,202 units/L), suggestive of hepatic failure triggered by infections and neutropenia that responded to G-CSF treatment. She is currently 7 years of age and continues to be on multiple daily injections of insulin, thyroxine replacement, 3-monthly pamidronate treatment, and multivitamin supplementation.

Wolcott-Rallison syndrome (WRS) (OMIM 226980) is an autosomal-recessive hereditary disease that causes non-autoimmune, insulin-deficient, permanent, early-onset diabetes.[1] Multiple epiphyseal dysplasia, growth retardation, acute liver failure, renal impairment, exocrine pancreas deficiency, intellectual deficits, neutropenia, and frequent infections are additional hallmarks of WRS. WRS is recognized as a common cause for persistent early-onset diabetes in children born to consanguineous parents.[2] Typical onset of type 1 diabetes is within the first 6 months of life (neonatal diabetes); however, onset may be delayed up to 30 months of age.[1-3]

WRS is caused by mutations in the EIF2AK3 gene, located on the short arm of the second chromosome encoding the transmembrane endoplasmic reticulum (ER) membrane, the PKR-like ER kinase (PERK).[4] PERK regulates the cellular response to ER stress and is essential for normal fetal and early neonatal β-cell proliferation, differentiation, and β-cell function. Hypoplastic pancreas, smaller-size Langerhans islets, and markedly reduced number of β-cells have been described in patients with WRS.[1,5] The severity and nature of the clinical course and manifestations of WRS show significant variability among patients and cannot be explained solely by the nature of the EIF2AK3 gene mutation.

WRS should be suspected in patients with a history of permanent neonatal/early-onset diabetes associated with skeletal dysplasia and/or episodes of acute liver failure. Type 1 diabetes is an obligate feature of WRS, and diabetic ketoacidosis at onset is not uncommon. In contrast to type 1A diabetes, the diabetes autoimmune panel is negative. Some of the distinctive clinical features of WRS might not be present at the onset of type 1 diabetes.

WRS is characterized by multiple epiphyseo-metaphyseal dysplasia and osteopenia that can manifest as multiple, frequent fractures. Vertebral abnormalities may lead to thoracic kyphosis and/or lumbar lordosis and chest deformities. Osteopenia and skeletal dysplasia have been attributed to loss of PERK expression in osteoblasts.[1]

Hepatic dysfunction, manifest in the form of elevated hepatic enzymes, hepatomegaly, and recurrent acute liver failure, is often triggered by inter-current illnesses such as mild upper respiratory tract infections and may be complicated by jaundice, hypoglycemia, and even coma in severe cases.[6] Hypo-glycemic episodes precede the diagnosis of diabetes and have been linked to impaired gluconeogenesis due to liver dysfunction.[5]

Our patient presented with classic WRS features, including neonatal type 1 diabetes, skeletal dysplasia, growth failure, recurrent neutropenia, and hepatic failure episodes. She had multiple episodes of transaminitis beginning from an early age, accompanied by neutropenia during most attacks. G-CSF for treat-ment of WRS-associated neutropenia has not been established as a standard of care and was used as an experimental treatment.

As shown in our case, short stature and skeletal dysplasia progressively develop and may be diagnosed after diabetes onset. Our patient had early grad-ual slowing of growth that progressed to severe short stature, osteoporosis, and impaired thyroid function at about 5 years of age. The underlying etiology of abnormal thyroid function in WRS is unclear.

WRS is a disease with a poor prognosis. Recurrent hepatic failure is a com-mon cause of mortality, and liver transplantation treatment has been explored in few WRS cases.[6] Close therapeutic monitoring is recommended given the tendency for frequent acute episodes of hypoglycemia, ketoacidosis, and acute multi-organ failure during intercurrent illness. Genetic counseling is recom-mended for extended consanguineous families with genetically diagnosed WRS.

COMMENTARY

Wolcott-Rallison syndrome is an autosomal-recessive disorder that is the most common genetic cause of neonatal diabetes. The vast majority of cases are diag-nosed within the first months of life. Mutations of the EIKF2AK3 gene that codes for PERK are responsible for the spectrum of symptoms. Ultimately, EIF2AK3 mutation screening confirms (or excludes) the WRS diagnosis. In terms of diabe-tes, close therapeutic monitoring is imperative because of the tendency for wide variations in the levels of glycemia. Patients develop frequent hypoglycemia and ketoacidosis. With this in mind, treatment with an insulin pump is frequently recommended, especially in small infants, to optimize the prevention of severe hypoglycemia. In contrast, this patient is doing reasonably well on multiple daily insulin injections.

Louis H. Philipson, MD, PhD, and Boris Draznin, MD, PhD

REFERENCES

1. Julier C, Nicolino M. Wolcott-Rallison syndrome. *Orphanet J Rare Dis* 2010;5:29

2. Rubio-Cabezas O, Patch AM, Minton JA, et al. Wolcott-Rallison syndrome is the most common genetic cause of permanent neonatal diabetes in consanguineous families. *J Clin Endocrinol Metab* 2009;94:4162–4170

3. Ozbek MN, Senée V, Aydemir S, et al. Wolcott-Rallison syndrome due to the same mutation (W522X) in EIF2AK3 in two unrelated families and review of the literature. *Pediatr Diabetes* 2010;11:279–285

4. Delepine M, Nicolino M, Barrett T, Golamaully M, Lathrop GM, Julier C. EIF2AK3, encoding translation initiation factor 2-alpha kinase 3, is mutated in patients with Wolcott-Rallison syndrome. *Nat Genet* 2000;25:406–409

5. Zhang W, Feng D, Li Y, Iida K, McGrath B, Cavener DR. PERK EIF2AK3 control of pancreatic beta cell differentiation and proliferation is required for postnatal glucose homeostasis. *Cell Metab* 2006;4:491–497

6. Tzakis AG, Nunnelley MJ, Tekin A, et al. Liver, pancreas and kidney transplantation for the treatment of Wolcott-Rallison syndrome. *Am J Transplant* 2015;15:565–567

Case 9

Glucose Intolerance Associated With ACTH-Dependent Cushing's Disease

Nitya K. Kumar, MD,[1] and Susan Spratt, MD[1]

A 67-year-old man with type 2 diabetes was admitted to the hospital for non-ST segment elevation myocardial infarction in the setting of worsening lower-extremity edema and hypokalemia. He was diagnosed with type 2 diabetes 20 years prior and had been well controlled, with a recent HbA$_{1c}$ of 6.5%. At the time of admission, he was on metformin and sulfonylurea therapy.

While admitted, he was noted to be severely hypertensive with systolic blood pressure in the 160s despite multiple agents and was persistently hypokalemic, with K$^+$ as low as 1.4 mmol/L. The severe refractory hypokalemia prompted a computed tomography (CT) scan of the abdomen with contrast because of concern for adrenal etiology. The scan revealed a benign-appearing right adrenal nodule. Coronary angiogram revealed <70% blockage, and he was started on dual anti-platelet therapy. The patient was discharged home with endocrinology follow-up.

Ten days later, he was found unconscious. Laboratory evaluation revealed the following:

Glucose: 303 mg/dL
Potassium: 2.2 mmol/L
HbA$_{1c}$: 8.2%
Renin: 0.31 ng/mL/h
Aldosterone: 1 ng/dL
AM cortisol: 55.8 ng/dL
Low-dose dexamethasone suppression test cortisol: 119.9 ng/dL with ACTH 293 pg/mL
High-dose 8-mg dexamethasone suppression test: baseline cortisol of 46.1 ng/dL and post-suppression level of 26.1 ng/dL
Urine free cortisol (UFC): 3,116 ng/24 h
Plasma metanephrines: 22 pg/mL
Plasma normetanephrines: 70 pg/mL

The patient was treated with intravenous insulin and regained consciousness. He reported that over the month before admission, he began

---

[1]Duke University Division of Endocrinology, Diabetes and Metabolism, Duke University School of Medicine, Durham, North Carolina.

DOI: 10.2337/9781580407663.09

noticing preprandial glucose values ranging from 180–250 mg/dL. He also noted mood changes with increased irritability along with proximal muscle weakness, facial plethora, polyuria, and weight loss of 10 lb over the last month.

The prevalence of diabetes in Cushing's disease (CD) has been reported to be between 20 and 45% of patients. Overall impairment in glucose metabolism among patients with CD is found in nearly 70% of cases.

Cortisol affects both glucose tolerance and insulin sensitivity. In the liver, cortisol exacerbates gluconeogenesis and hepatic glucose output, both directly and indirectly. Chronic glucocorticoid exposure causes liver insulin resistance, weakening the inhibitory effect of insulin on hepatic glucose release, as well as skeletal muscle insulin resistance with decreasing glucose uptake. Excess cortisol also affects growth hormone levels, leading to an increase in visceral fat and insulin resistance.[1] Cortisol excess in patients with CD leads to increased appetite and other central effects, as well as pancreatic β-cell dysfunction.[2]

Repeat CT of the abdomen/pelvis without contrast confirmed a lipid-rich right adrenal adenoma that measured 8 HU. Pituitary magnetic resonance imaging was negative for adenoma. Results of inferior petrosal sinus (IPS) sampling are shown below (Table 9.1). Corticorelin was given after baseline measurements were taken. Although the patient's IPS sampling did not quite meet the diagnostic cutoff of 3:1 post-corticorelin, typically used for supporting a pituitary etiology of CD, the left IPS ACTH levels rose at 5 min and yielded a ratio of 2.58 compared to the peripheral/femoral region. Positron emission tomography scan was negative for somatostatin receptor avid neoplasm.

The patient continued to have poorly controlled blood pressure, hypokalemia, and hyperglycemia, so he was started on ketoconazole with dose adjusted to 600 mg daily, along with an ACE inhibitor, spironolactone, and potassium supplements. For diabetes management, he was started on lispro insulin corrections while his glycemia ranged from 200 to in the 300s, with fasting glucose as high as 270 mg/dL. His regimen was eventually modified to include glargine 20 units daily and lispro 15 units with meals, in addition to metformin 2 g daily. Fasting glucose improved to the 90s, with preprandial glucose levels <130 mg/dL. Despite treatment for 10 days with ketoconazole and improvement in 24-h UFC to 764 ng, the hypokalemia

Table 9.1—IPS sampling results

ACTH (units)	Baseline	3 min	5 min	10 min	15 min
Femoral	51	64	67	68	61
Left IPS	70	140	173	149	69
Right IPS	66	69	73	90	82, 80

persisted with potassium as low as 2.3 mmol/L while on an ACE inhibitor and spironolactone. His dose of ketoconazole was eventually increased to a maximum of 1,200 mg daily, with improvement in 24-h UFC to 35 ng.

Adrenal steroidogenesis inhibitors are a mainstay of medical therapy in CD and have been shown to improve glycemic control in CD.[3] Ketoconazole inhibits steroidogenesis, thereby reducing cortisol synthesis by blocking numerous enzymes in the steroid pathway, including 11-β-hydroxylase and 17-α-hydroxylase. Cortisol excess can be rapidly controlled, but because of the "escape phenomenon," higher doses may be needed long term for successful maintenance.

A French retrospective multicenter study illustrated the efficacy of ketoconazole monotherapy on glycemic control in CD, defined by one or more of the following: a decrease in insulin dose >10%, a decrease in the number of antidiabetic drugs, and/or an improvement of HbA_{1c} of >0.5% without addition of other antidiabetic drugs. In the 200 patients examined, over 30% of patients had diabetes before treatment. Ketoconazole normalized UFC levels in almost 50% of patients, with another 25% of patients having at least a 50% decrease. Of the 20%[2] who received ketoconazole as presurgical treatment, 50% had improvement in their diabetes over a mean period of 4 months on a mean final dose of 755 mg/day. In patients on long-term treatment with ketoconazole (over 24 months), 50% had improvement in diabetes at their final follow-up visit, along with over 87% having improvement in hypokalemia.[3]

With regards to glycemic treatment, in addition to starting targeted medical therapy to reduce cortisol levels, patients should be managed similar to individuals with type 2 diabetes.[2] In our patient, weight-based insulin dosing at ~0.6 units/kg along with metformin was used to achieve glycemic control while being initiated on ketoconazole. In addition to the known glycemic benefits of metformin, recent studies in mouse models suggest that metformin may actually have direct antitumor activity against pituitary corticotroph tumors as well as ACTH secretion.[4]

Higher prandial insulin requirements, as seen in our patient, are not surprising given the predominant effect of steroids on prandial glycemia. For this reason, it is also recommended that screening for steroid-induced diabetes be done using postprandial glucose determinants and/or HbA_{1c} rather than fasting glucose or glucose tolerance testing.[5]

Although imaging was unremarkable, given the IPS sampling results, there was a concern for an intraglandular ACTH-producing microadenoma. The patient was taken for pituitary exploration. No discrete adenoma was seen and the left side of the pituitary gland was removed. Serum cortisol on postoperative day (POD) 1 improved to 50 ng/dL and to 21 ng/dL on POD 2, with ACTH of 62 pg/mL while on ketoconazole. Random cortisol eventually fell to 15 ng/dL with ACTH of 54 pg/mL.

Several months later, repeat imaging of the pituitary showed expected postoperative changes with 25% of the left side of the pituitary gland removed, and the remainder of the gland and stalk was intact and normal without evidence of tumor. Potassium had normalized and his ketoconazole

dose was reduced to **800 mg daily**. He remained on spironolactone and potassium supplements. His glargine dose was reduced to **15 units daily** and prandial coverage could be managed with correction scale only.

COMMENTARY

Interference of glucocorticoids with glycemic control is one of the most prevalent and difficult-to-address medical problems in patients with diabetes. Endogenous excess of glucocorticoids can be as detrimental (if not more so) than exogenous steroids prescribed for a variety of medical conditions. Impaired glucose tolerance has long been described as one of the main features of endogenous glucocorticoid excess.

The case presented by Drs. Kumar and Spratt also illustrates the therapeutic dilemma in treatment of patients with CD and overt diabetes. This complex and interesting patient was treated with both partial hypophysectomy and ketoconazole with moderate improvement in his hypercortisolemia. Nevertheless, the patient required moderate doses of insulin on the background of metformin that were eventually reduced to 15 units glargine and corrections with a short-acting insulin.

Certainly, reductions in the levels of cortisol and initiation and maintenance of insulin therapy are the major factors in improvement of this patient's glycemia. One would hope his remission of CD is long-lasting.

Boris Draznin, MD, PhD

REFERENCES

1. Barbot M, Ceccato F, Scaroni C. Diabetes mellitus secondary to Cushing's disease. *Front Endocrinol (Lausanne)* 2018;9:284

2. Colao A, De Block C, Gaztambide MS, Kumar S, Seufert J, Casanueva FF. Managing hyperglycemia in patients with Cushing's disease treated with pasireotide: medical expert recommendations. *Pituitary* 2014;17:180–186

3. Castinetti F, Guignat L, Giraud P, et al. Ketoconazole in Cushing's disease: is it worth a try? *J Clin Endocrinol Metab* 2014;99:1623–1630

4. Jin K, Ruan L, Pu J, et al. Metformin suppresses growth and adrenocorticotrophic hormone secretion in mouse pituitary corticotroph tumor AtT20cells. *Mol Cell Endocrinol* 2018;478:53–61

5. Tamez-Perez HE, Quintanilla-Flores DL, Rodriguez-Gutierrez R, Gonzalez-Gonzalez JG, Tamez-Pena AL. Steroid hyperglycemia: prevalence, early detection and therapeutic recommendations: a narrative review. *World J Diabetes* 2015;6:1073–1081

Case 10

Maturity-Onset Diabetes of the Young (MODY) Misdiagnosis as Steroid-Induced Diabetes

GHADA ELSHIMY, MD,[1] AND RICARDO CORREA, MD, EdD, FACP, FACE, FAPCR, CMQ[1]

A 24-year-old male with a past medical history of eosinophilic vasculitis diagnosed in 2015 had been on intermittent courses of high-dose steroids when he presented to an outside emergency department in 2016 with polyuria, polydipsia, blurry vision, elevated blood glucose, and mild ketones in the urine with an eosinophilic vasculitis flare. He was diagnosed with steroid-induced hyperglycemia and discharged home on metformin 1,000 mg twice daily. His blood glucose was subsequently controlled on metformin for almost 1 year. However, in 2017, despite discontinuation of the steroids, his blood glucose trended upward with most of the readings in the 300–400 mg/dL range; therefore, he was started on glargine 10 units daily and aspart correctional scale for meals (1 unit of aspart for every 50 mg/dL of blood glucose above 150 mg/dL). He had multiple hypoglycemic episodes on that regimen. In 2018, the patient was referred to our endocrine clinic for further evaluation. On questioning, the patient stated that there was no family history of diabetes or autoimmune diseases. He also mentioned that his weight had not changed since diagnosis.

On physical examination, the patient's blood pressure was 114/73 mmHg and pulse rate was 60 beats/min. His height was 75 inches (190.2 cm) and weight was 169.6 lb (77.4 kg) (BMI 21 kg/m²). Findings from the neurological and physical examinations were normal. No acanthosis nigricans or signs of lipodystrophy were noticed on skin examination. Laboratory test results showed HbA$_{1c}$ of 8.4% with a fasting blood glucose level of 180 mg/dL. The remaining blood work did not show any significant abnormalities (Table 10.1). Further testing included C-peptide of 2.15 ng/mL when the blood glucose was 137 mg/dL, indicating pancreatic reserve. Additionally, islet cell antibodies and anti-GAD65 antibodies were negative. Given the age of the patient, BMI, and the laboratory test results, there was high suspicion for maturity-onset diabetes of the young (MODY). The patient was then referred for genetic testing and started on glipizide 5 mg twice daily while waiting for the genetic results to come back. After 2 weeks of glipizide, insulin was discontinued. Genetic testing came back positive for glucokinase mutation (MODY-2, exon 2 c.182A>C p.Tyr61Ser). Blood glucose was stable on only one glucose-lowering medication, with no hypoglycemic episodes.

[1]Division of Endocrinology, University of Arizona College of Medicine, Phoenix, Arizona.

DOI: 10.2337/9781580407663.10

Table 10.1—Summary of laboratory results

Laboratory test	Results	References
HbA$_{1c}$, %	8.4	4–6
C-peptide, ng/mL	2.15	0.8–3.85
Fasting blood glucose, mg/dL	137	74–106
Blood urea nitrogen, mg/dL	12	7–20
Creatinine, mg/dL	0.92 mg/dL	0.52–1.25
Glomerular filtration rate	>60	>60
Albumin-to-creatinine ratio, mg/g	7.4	≤30
Total cholesterol, mg/dL	187	<200
Triglyceride, mg/dL	198	<150
LDL, g/dL	112	<130
HDL, mg/dL	36	30–60

MODY is an autosomal-dominant familial diabetes that was first reported in 1974.[1] MODY is the most common form of monogenic diabetes. It accounts for an estimated 1–2% of diabetes. Unfortunately, it is often misdiagnosed as type 1 diabetes or sometimes as type 2 diabetes. The diagnostic criteria set forth in the practice guidelines for MODY in 2008 include the age of onset before 25 years old with the absence of β-cell autoantibodies (anti-GAD65, anti–islet cell, Zinc transporter, and others) and preserved β-cell function. Additional criteria include the presence of diabetes in two consecutive generations. Sustained endogenous insulin secretion is indicated by either the presence of a serum C-peptide level >200 pmol/L, even after 3 years of insulin treatment or the lack of need for insulin treatment.[2] Molecular methods for the diagnosis of MODY were first introduced after the 1990s and, currently, mutations in at least 14 different genes have been associated with MODY.[2] To improve the prognosis of MODY, the early identification of the affected subjects is essential. Currently, specific molecular analyses are available to predict the clinical disease course and offer the most appropriate treatment.[3] We present a patient who was initially misdiagnosed as having steroid-induced diabetes; however, upon referral to endocrinology, MODY-2 was confirmed, and the patient had an excellent response to sulfonylurea treatment.

The correct determination of the MODY subtype is essential to determine the appropriate treatment and prognosis. The six genes encoding major factors are hepatocyte nuclear factor (HNF)-4α, glucokinase (GCK), HNF1α, pancreatic and duodenal homeobox 1 (PDX1), HNF1β, and neurogenic differentiation 1 (NEUROD1), which correspond to MODY subtypes 1–6, respectively.[2] GCK (MODY-2) and HNF1α (MODY-3) are the most common identified mutations. Treatment is variable according to the subtype. Some patients are controlled with dietary modification only. However, medical treatment may be needed in other patients, including either oral antidiabetic medications (sulfonylureas) and/or insulin. The selection of appropriate treatments for these patients is important to improve their quality of life and avoid hypoglycemic episodes.[3]

MODY-1 is due to a mutation in HNF4α on chromosome 20 leading to a genetic defect in insulin secretion. It typically presents in adolescence. The disease is progressive but has a good response to sulfonylureas (some patients may require insulin later on). These patients can develop micro- and macrovascular complications.[3] MODY-2 is due to a mutation in GCK on chromosome 7 leading to an insulin secretory defect. GCK phosphorylates glucose to glucose-6-phosphate and acts as a glucose sensor. A mutation in this gene results in a higher threshold for glucose-stimulated insulin secretion. This was the case for our patient. Unlike MODY-1, MODY-2 is not associated with vascular complications. Hyperglycemia is usually mild, stable, and often controlled with diet.[4] MODY-3 is due to a mutation in the HNF1α gene on chromosome 12, leading to glucosuria (due to lowering of the renal threshold for glucose reabsorption) with abnormal insulin secretion, but the exact mechanism is unclear. These patients have similar clinical phenotypes as the HNF4α mutation.[5]

Given the heterogeneity of presentations of diabetes, the physician should suspect MODY when classic clinical manifestations do not fit the criteria for either type 1 or type 2 diabetes. When there is clinical suspicion for atypical diabetes, referral for genetic testing is an essential step in confirming the diagnosis and establishing adequate treatment in these patients.

COMMENTARY

MODY is the most common form of monogenic diabetes and is well recognized in clinical practice. It is classified as atypical diabetes to be distinguished from both type 1 and type 2 diabetes. The term was coined by Tattersall and Fajans in 1974 and, since that time, many mutations corresponding to distinct clinical presentations have been identified. The authors correctly point out that a high index of suspicion coupled with genetic testing help astute clinicians arrive at the correct diagnosis and treatment. This case is an important illustration of a rational approach to patients with diabetes who present with an atypical clinical course. Genetic confirmation of the GCK mutation was critical to arrive at the correct diagnosis.

Boris Draznin, MD, PhD

REFERENCES

1. Tattersall RB. Mild familial diabetes with dominant inheritance. *Q J Med* 1974;43:339–357

2. Urakami T. Maturity-onset diabetes of the young (MODY): current perspectives on diagnosis and treatment. *Diabetes Metab Syndr Obes* 2019;12:1047–1056

3. Hattersley AT, Greeley SA, Polak M, et al. ISPAD clinical practice consensus guidelines 2018: the diagnosis and management of monogenic diabetes in children and adolescents. *Pediatr Diabetes* 2018;19:47–63

4. Froguel P, Zouali H, Vionnet N, et al. Familial hyperglycemia due to mutations in glucokinase: definition of a subtype of diabetes mellitus. *N Engl J Med* 1993;328:697

5. Yamagata K, Oda N, Kaisaki PJ, et al. Mutations in the hepatocyte nuclear factor-1alpha gene in maturity-onset diabetes of the young (MODY3). *Nature* 1996;384:455

Part 2

Diabetic Ketoacidosis (DKA) and Euglycemic DKA

Case 11

A Case of Histiocytosis-Lymphadenopathy Plus Syndrome Due to a Novel Mutation in the *SLC29A3* Gene and Presentation With Diabetic Ketoacidosis

Gül Yeşiltepe-Mutlu, MD,[1] Mehmet N. Özbek, MD,[2] and Eda Cengiz, MD, MHS, FAAP[3,4]

An 11-and-a-half-year-old boy of Kurdish descent born to consanguineous parents presented to our clinic with polydypsia, polyuria, and weight loss. His prenatal and natal medical history was unremarkable. His prior medical history was significant for hearing loss at 2 years of age and surgical repair of omphalocele. He was reported to have low school performance and was enrolled in a special education class. There was a family history of type 2 diabetes diagnosed in his father, maternal grandmother, and paternal grandmother in their late 40s.

Physical examination revealed a height of 4.1 ft (–2.8 standard deviation score [SDS]) and a weight of 55.1 lb (–2.6 SDS), indicative of growth retardation. He had dysmorphic features including a triangular face and enlarged ears and was wearing a hearing aid. There was a hyperpigmented area measuring 1.5 × 2.4 inches (4 × 6 cm) on the inner surface of his thighs and calves (Figure 11.1). The rest of the physical exam findings were unremarkable.

Laboratory tests revealed a blood glucose level of 800 mg/dL and a pH of 7.28, indicative of mild diabetic ketoacidosis (DKA). HbA$_{1c}$ level was 12.4%. Serum C-peptide level was 0.29 ng/mL. Serum anti-GAD antibody was positive at 26.9 units/mL (<5 IU/mL). The patient had an elevated erythrocyte sedimentation rate (ESR) with normal hemoglobin and normal liver enzymes. Thyroid function tests and serum cortisol level were in the normal range. The bone age X-ray result assessed by the Greulich-Pyle method was consistent with a bone age delay of 24 months. The patient was treated with intravenous (IV) insulin drip and IV fluids, and he was transitioned to multiple daily basal-bolus insulin injections after the DKA resolved. Genetic testing was performed to determine the possibility of a syndromic cause (specifically H syndrome) for his hearing loss and hyperpigmented skin

[1]Division of Pediatric Endocrinology and Diabetes, Koç University School of Medicine, İstanbul, Turkey. [2]Gazi Yasargil Training and Research Hospital Clinics of Pediatric Endocrinology, Diyarbakır, Turkey. [3]Division of Pediatric Endocrinology and Diabetes, Yale School of Medicine, New Haven, Connecticut. [4]Visiting Professor, Bahcesehir University, Istanbul, Turkey.

DOI: 10.2337/9781580407663.11

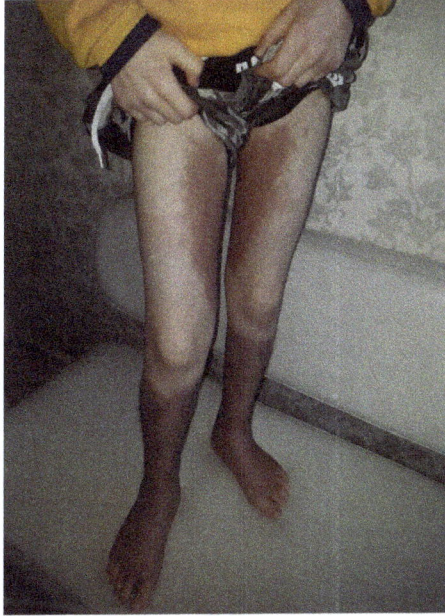

Figure 11.1—Symmetrical hyperpigmented indurated plaques over medial aspect of the lower extremities.

markings in the setting of parental consanguinity. The mutation analysis of the *SLC29A3* gene revealed a novel homozygous mutation c.1013_1013delG (p.Gly338AlafsTer67) in exon 6, confirming the diagnosis of H syndrome.

Histiocytosis-lymphadenopathy plus (HLP) syndrome (OMIM 602782) is an autosomal-recessive disorder that is caused by homozygous or compound heterozygous mutation in the SLC29A3 gene. The SLC29A3 gene is located on chromosome 10q22 and encodes hENT3, a nucleoside transporter that plays a significant role in macrophage apoptotic cell clearance. Mice lacking ENT3 have been shown to develop macrophage-dominated histiocytosis.[1]

Multiple histiocytic disorders have been classified under the HLP syndrome, which includes H syndrome, pigmented hypertrichosis with insulin-dependent diabetes (PHID), Faisalabad histiocytosis, and familial Rosai-Dorfman disease. More recently, these disorders have been grouped under the same entity termed H syndrome given the overlapping clinical features and shared genetic etiology.

H syndrome is named for a collection of clinical symptoms characterized by cutaneous **h**yperpigmentation, **h**ypertrichosis, **h**epatosplenomegaly, **h**eart anomalies, **h**earing loss, **h**ypogonadism, short stature (**h**eight), and **h**yperglycemia due to type 1 diabetes. The clinical findings are known to be widely variable and may also include flexion contractures of fingers and toes, hallux valgus, genital swelling, episcleritis, exophthalmos, lymphadenopathy (generalized or localized), or gastrointestinal and bone marrow abnormalities.[2] Interstitial histiocytic infiltration has been shown in histology of skin lesions, enlarged lymph nodes, and nasal mucosa.[2]

Herein, we describe a case of H syndrome with new-onset type 1 diabetes. The differential diagnosis during admission included thiamine-responsive megaloblastic anemia (TRMA) syndrome and Wolfram syndrome given that our patient had type 1 diabetes and sensorineural hearing impairment at the time of presentation. TRMA syndrome was ruled out by absence of anemia, and Wolfram syndrome was ruled out based on the absence of the usual characteristic features of the syndrome (i.e., diabetes insipidus, optic nerve atrophy, and neurodegeneration). More importantly, our patient had positive anti-GAD antibodies, which are negative in both TRMA and Wolfram syndromes.

Findings on skin examination are pathognomonic for H syndrome. These skin manifestations are characterized by patches of hyperpigmentation commonly observed on the lower extremities. Pigmented areas with hypertrichosis have been described in patients with the PHID that is classified under the H syndrome spectrum.[3]

Table 11.1—Clinical characteristics and presentation of H syndrome patients with type 1 diabetes

	Present Case	Ref. 1	Ref. 2	Ref. 3	Ref. 3	Ref. 3	Ref. 4	Ref. 5
Sex	Male	Female	Female	Female	Female	Female	Male	Female
Age at H syndrome diagnosis (years)	11.5	19	10	8	20	15	22	<1
Age at onset of diabetes symptoms (years)	11.5	Unknown	16	Unknown	Unknown	Unknown	22	4
Presentation at the diagnosis	DKA	DKA	Hyperglycemia Ketonemia	Hyperglycemia	Unknown	Unknown	DKA	Unknown
Diabetes autoantibody status	Anti-GAD positive, anti-insulin negative, anti-ICA negative	Unknown	Anti-GAD positive, anti-insulin negative, anti-ICA negative	Anti-GAD positive, anti-insulin positive, anti-ICA positive	Anti-GAD positive, anti-ICA negative	Anti-GAD positive, anti-ICA negative	Anti-GAD negative	Anti-GAD negative, anti-ICA negative
Other autoimmune antibodies, inflammatory markers	Anti-TTG thyroid antibodies negative, elevated CRP	Unknown	Anti-endomysium positive, anti-TTG positive, thyroid antibodies negative, elevated ESR and CRP	Anti-endomysium positive	Elevated ESR and CRP	Elevated ESR and CRP	Unknown	Persistently high CRP and ESR
Lipoatrophy	No		Yes					Yes

Anti-TTG, anti-transglutaminase IgA; CRP, C-reactive protein; ICA, islet cell antibody.

The constellation of findings including the hyperpigmented cutaneous lesions on lower extremities (albeit without hypertrichosis), severe short stature, and sensorineural hearing impairment in the setting of type 1 diabetes were highly suggestive of H syndrome for our patient. The diagnosis was confirmed by the genetic testing showing a novel mutation in the SLC29A3 gene.

Histiocytosis and tissue damage mediated by accumulation of histiocytes are common features of H syndrome spectrum disorders that manifest in different parts of the body. Hallux valgus, hepatosplenomegaly, lymphadenopathy, flexion contractures in the joints, and cardiac anomalies that were described in other published cases with H syndrome were not present in our patient. Although our patient had dysmorphic facial findings, none of them were congruent with the previously described typical features of H syndrome (i.e., bilateral ptosis, epicanthal folds, and low-set ears).

Type 1 diabetes is reported as being present in up to 23% of individuals with H syndrome.[2] The clinical and biochemical findings of these cases are summarized in Table 11.1. In H syndrome, diabetes is thought to develop via an inflammatory mechanism that destroys pancreatic β-cells. Another possible mechanism is that mutation of SLC29A3-coded hENT3 disrupts interaction with the insulin-signaling pathway, resulting in impaired insulin secretion.[3]

Ref. 5	Ref. 6	Ref. 7	Ref. 7	Ref. 7	Ref. 8	Ref. 9	Ref. 10	Ref. 10	Ref. 11
Female	Female	Male	Male	Male	Female	Male	Male	Male	Female
12	5	15	11	12	11	17	6	21	20.5
12	5	15	11	12	11	14	1.5	10	1.5
Unknown	Unknown	DKA	Unknown	Unknown	Hyperglycemia Ketonuria	Unknown	Unknown	Unknown	Unknown
Anti-GAD negative, anti-ICA negative	Anti-GAD positive, anti-ICA positive	Anti-GAD positive	Anti ICA negative	Unknown	Unknown	Unknown	Unknown	Unknown	Unknown
Persistently high CRP and ESR	Elevated ESR and CRP	Unknown	Elevated ESR and CRP	Unknown	Elevated ESR and CRP	Unknown	Unknown	Persistently high CRP and ESR	Unknown
Yes	Yes	Yes		Yes	Unknown	Unknown	Unknown		No

The presence of diabetes-related autoantibodies in some cases, including our patient, suggests the possibility of an autoimmune cause.

The timing and presentation of diabetes in H syndrome is variable. Patients present in DKA or with hyperglycemia without ketosis after a gradual asymptomatic progressive course with anti-GAD positivity and impaired glucose tolerance.[4]

In conclusion, H syndrome is a rare genetic disease with a pattern of signs and symptoms that can vary, even within the same family. This syndrome should be considered in the differential diagnosis of patients who present with cutaneous hyperpigmentation, sensorineural hearing loss, and type 1 diabetes.

COMMENTARY

The authors present a young patient with physical manifestations suggestive of a syndromic cause of his insulin-deficient diabetes and presentation with DKA. H syndrome, or histiocytosis-lymphadenopathy plus syndrome, is one of the described rare genetic causes of insulin-deficient diabetes. These disorders are more likely to be encountered in the pediatric-age population, where there needs to be a high index of suspicion for atypical causes for new-onset type 1 diabetes, as illustrated in this case. The early-onset of hearing loss, hyperpigmented skin lesions, and dysmorphic features raised consideration for genetic testing in this child. Given that the authors report that 23% of individuals with this syndrome develop type 1 diabetes, regular monitoring of blood glucose together with educating caregivers in signs and symptoms of hyperglycemia could possibly allow diagnosis before presentation with DKA.

Mary Korytkowski, MD

REFERENCES

1. Molho-Pessach V, Lerer I, Abeliovich D, et al. The H syndrome is caused by mutations in the nucleoside transporter hENT3. *Am J Hum Genet* 2008;83:529–534

2. Molho-Pessach V, Ramot Y, Camille F, et al. The H syndrome: the first 79 patients. *J Am Acad Dermatol* 2014;70:80–88

3. Cliffe ST, Kramer JM, Hussain K, et al. SLC29A3 gene is mutated in pigmented hypertrichosis with insulin-dependent diabetes mellitus syndrome and interacts with the insulin signaling pathway. *Hum Mol Genet* 2009;18: 2257–2265

4. Ozlu C, Yesiltepe Mutlu G, Hatun S. A Turkish girl with H syndrome: stunted growth and development of autoimmune insulin dependent diabetes mellitus in the 6th year of diagnosis. *J Pediatr Endocrinol Metab* 2019;32:89–93. doi:10.1515/jpem-2018-0380

Case 12

Acromegaly Presenting With Diabetic Ketoacidosis

Ritika Verma, MD,[1] Kiet Huynh, BS,[1] Rajani Gundluru, MD,[2] Michael J. Gardner, MD,[2] and James Sowers, MD[2]

We present a 31-year-old male without any comorbidities who presented to the emergency room (ER) with a 2-week history of polyuria, polydipsia, constipation, and fatigue. He also reported a weight loss of 40 lb over the last 3 months. During the interview, he mentioned having oily skin and acne all of his life. He denied palpitations, hyperhidrosis, or difficulty with sexual activity. Physical exam was striking for frontal bossing, prognathism, hypertrichosis, and large hands and feet, suggesting acromegaly. No acanthosis nigricans or acrochordons was noted. Initial lab work revealed the following: blood glucose 241 mg/dL, serum bicarbonate 12 mEq/L, anion gap 31, β-hydroxybutyrate >8 mmol/L, ketonuria on urinalysis, and HbA_{1c} of 13.1%. Islet cell anti-GAD antibodies were negative.

With a working diagnosis of diabetic ketoacidosis (DKA) and acromegaly, further workup was done. An impaired fasting glucose (IGF)-1 level was increased at 1,094 ng/mL. Magnetic resonance imaging of the pituitary demonstrated a 2.1 × 1.3 × 2.1 cm enhancing sellar mass confirming a pituitary macro-adenoma and acromegaly.

He was initially treated with an intravenous insulin infusion, followed by transition to a subcutaneous regimen of insulin glargine 50 units every 12 h and meal coverage with insulin (lispro) using an insulin:carbohydrate ratio of 1:3. A correction factor of 1 additional unit of lispro for each 50 mg/dL increment in blood glucose >150 mg/dL was also prescribed. The patient underwent a trans-sphenoidal pituitary resection after which his insulin requirements gradually decreased. He was titrated off of insulin about 1 month later. His HbA_{1c} soon normalized at 5.7%.

At a 3-month follow-up visit, he had an elevated IGF (1,196 ng/mL) and growth hormone level (11.49 ng/mL). Nevertheless, his HbA_{1c} continued to be normal at 5.7%, and he has not required any anti-diabetic treatment since his surgery. A thin band of residual tumor along the right lateral sella

[1]Internal Medicine, University of Missouri, Columbia, Missouri. [2]Endocrinology and Diabetes Division, University of Missouri School of Medicine, Columbia, Missouri.

DOI: 10.2337/9781580407663.12

was confirmed on repeat imaging and is further being managed with a combination of octreotide and stereotactic radiotherapy.

While diabetes is seen in ~10–25% of patients presenting with acromegaly, DKA is rare.[1] HbA_{1c} has been shown to have a direct linear relationship with IGF-1 levels and associated insulin resistance in acromegalic patients, but DKA in this condition occurs as a result of relative insulin deficiency. Diabetes in these patients often resolves with curative treatment of the primary disease and normalization of IGF-1 levels. Our patient presented to the ER with DKA without a prior diagnosis of acromegaly or diabetes. The last reported case of acromegaly presenting as DKA was in 2017.

DKA is a rare complication of acromegaly,[1,2] and the fact that DKA was the initial presenting feature in our patient makes the case unique. While insulin resistance is the most common cause of diabetes in acromegaly, DKA is attributed to glucotoxicity and lipotoxicity leading to β-cell dysfunction and is typically reversible with initiating strategies to improve glycemic control.[1,2] DKA develops from a severe insulin deficiency, absolute or relative, in combination with an excess of the counter-regulatory hormones glucagon, catecholamines, cortisol, and growth hormone (GH)/IGF-1,[3] as in this case.

Another fascinating aspect of our case came forward during his clinic follow-up. Almost all reported cases of diabetes associated with acromegaly show a direct linear relationship between GH/IGF-1 levels and HbA_{1c}.[3] However, while workup for a possible residual tumor revealed high IGF-1 and GH levels, our patient's HbA_{1c} remained in the normal range despite discontinuation

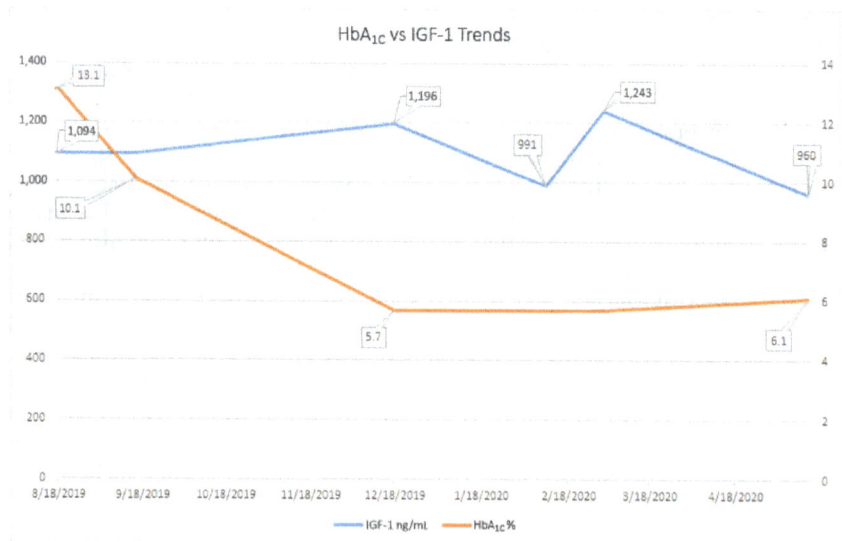

Figure 12.1 — IGF-1 and HbA_{1c} levels since diagnosis.

of insulin therapy (5.7 and 6.1%, 3 and 8 months post-resection, respectively) (Figure 12.1). An ongoing follow-up period that includes monitoring of glycemic control is necessary to avoid recurrent DKA.

COMMENTARY

DKA is a rare presenting feature of acromegaly, but cases similar to this patient have been reported. This case illustrates that individuals with undiagnosed acromegaly are not only at risk for abnormal glucose tolerance that often presents as type 2 diabetes, but are also at risk for more severe degrees of hyperglycemia. The abnormal glucose tolerance that occurs in these patients is usually attributed to growth hormone–mediated insulin resistance. When insulin resistance is prolonged or severe, hyperglycemia together with elevations in free fatty acids result in impaired insulin secretion that in turn can precipitate acute metabolic decompensation. As the authors point out, a linear relationship has been reported between IGF-1 and HbA_{1c} levels; however, the fact that his HbA_{1c} level remains in a pre-diabetes range despite persistent elevations in IGF-1 levels suggests that there are other factors contributing to hyperglycemia in these patients. Of note, hyperglycemia and DKA can also occur with use of the somatostatin analogs that are often used either for treating acromegaly as primary therapy or when surgery does not result in normalization of growth hormone and IGF-1 levels. This patient warrants ongoing surveillance during therapy of his now-diagnosed acromegaly.

Mary Korytkowski, MD

REFERENCES

1. Chen Y-L, Wei C-P, Lee C-C-, Chang T-C. Diabetic ketoacidosis in a patient with acromegaly. *J Formo Med Assoc* 106;2007:788–791. https://doi.org/10.1016/S0929-6646(08)60042-X

2. Reddy R, Hope S, Wass J. Acromegaly. *BMJ* 2010;341:c4189. https://doi.org/10.1136/bmj.c4189

3. Palakawong P, Arakaki R. Diabetic ketoacidosis in acromegaly: a case report. Endoc Pract 2012 Nov 27:1–15. https://doi.org/10.4158/EP12189.CR

4. Alberti KGMM, Christensen MJ, Iversen J, Ørskov H. Role of glucagon and other hormones in development of diabetic ketoacidosis. *Lancet* 1975;1: 1307–1311. https://doi.org/10.1016/S0140-6736(75)92315-6

5. Chanson P, Salenave S, Kamenicky P. Acromegaly. In *Handbook of Clinical Neurology*. Fliers E, Korbonits M, Romijn JA, Eds. Elsevier, 2014, p. 197–219. https://doi.org/10.1016/B978-0-444-59602-4.00014-9

Case 13

Rapid-Onset Type 1 Diabetes and Ketoacidosis

Deepthi Rimmalapudi, MD,[1] and Eli Ipp, MD[1]

A 54-year-old Hispanic male presented to the emergency department with a 2-day history of nausea, vomiting, polydipsia, and generalized weakness. He was found to be in severe diabetic ketoacidosis with serum glucose of 1,062 mg/dL, pH of 6.84, HCO_3 of 5 mmol/L, anion gap of 25, and β-hydroxybutyrate of 11 mmol/L. He denied a previous history of diabetes, but was told 1 year earlier that he had prediabetes and was treated with diet. He was managed in the intensive care unit (ICU) with fluid and electrolyte resuscitation and insulin infusion and was switched to a basal-bolus insulin regimen once ketoacidosis resolved. His HbA_{1c} was 8% on admission (yet fasting plasma glucose was 106 mg/dL 1 month earlier), with C-peptide of 0.05 nmol/L, anti-GAD >250 IU/mL, and negative anti-insulin and anti–IA-2 antibodies. The patient was diagnosed with type 1 diabetes, and he remains insulin-dependent to date.

This rapid development and presentation of type 1 diabetes and severe ketoacidosis with extremely high serum glucose despite relatively mild HbA_{1c} elevation, and after a slightly abnormal fasting glucose 1 month earlier, is distinctly unusual except when understood in the context of key additional information in the history.

Three days before admission, the patient received a second cycle of systemic therapy with nivolumab and ipilimumab for stage IV clear cell carcinoma after removal of the right kidney.

The time course suggests a different diagnosis: rapid-onset, immune checkpoint inhibitor (ICI) insulinopenic diabetes. There is clear evidence to implicate the checkpoint inhibitor therapy in the etiology of both autoimmune diabetes and its rapid onset.

ICIs are increasingly being used for management of an expanding and broad range of malignancies. ICIs are used to restore deficient intrinsic anti-tumor immune responses by blocking immune receptors, including the cytotoxic T-lymphocyte antigen-4 (CTLA-4), the programmed cell death

[1]Lundquist Research Institute at Harbor-UCLA Medical Center, Torrance, California.

 DOI: 10.2337/9781580407663.13

receptor-1 (PD-1), or its ligand, PD-L1. ICIs are known to cause immune-related adverse events, commonly affecting the skin, gastrointestinal tract, liver, and endocrine system.

Endocrinopathies caused by ICIs are often irreversible. Although it is the pituitary, thyroid, and adrenal glands that are typically affected, the endocrine pancreas can also be a target and leads to rapid onset of insulin-dependent diabetes. In this patient with autoimmune diabetes, a combination of PD-1 and CTLA-4 inhibitor was used to treat his clear cell carcinoma of the kidney.

PD-1 is a cell surface receptor expressed on chronically activated CD8+ T-cells. It binds with its ligands PD-L1 and PD-L2, which are expressed on antigen-presenting cells (APCs) and tumor cells, negatively regulating effector T-cell responses. CD28 is a costimulatory molecule expressed on naive and regulatory T-cells, and its binding to CD80 or CD86 on APCs causes T-cell activation. CTLA-4 binds to CD28 and prevents this immune response. Monoclonal antibodies to PD-1, PD-L1, or CTLA-4 effectively negate these checkpoints of immune regulation and boost anti-tumor immunity.[1] However, these processes also play a key role in maintaining tolerance to self-antigens, and any disruption can lead to autoimmune disorders.

In nonobese diabetic (NOD) mice, PD-1 and PD-L1 have been shown to be important in the regulation of autoimmune diabetes. Exposure to blocking antibodies to PD-1 or PD-L1 result in accelerated development of diabetes in NOD mice at all ages, but is more pronounced in older mice. In contrast, CTLA-4 inhibition causes diabetes only in neonatal mice. Based on studies with lymphocyte-deficient mice, both CD4+ and CD8+ positive T-cells but not B-cells are critical for the autoimmune response. Two steps have been documented: an initial priming of T-cells in the pancreatic lymph nodes followed by infiltration and destruction of islet cells. PD-1/PD-L1 inhibitors augment the immune response in both steps.[2]

In humans, genetic polymorphisms and mutations in PD-1/PD-L1 and CTLA-4 alleles were found to be associated with Hashimoto's thyroiditis, Graves' disease, type 2 diabetes, and Addison's disease.[1] Histologic examination of pancreatic tissue in one patient showed extensive CD8+ T-cell infiltration and islet cell destruction, showing similarity to mouse models.[3]

Studies of HLA haplotypes suggest that the ICI-associated diabetes occurs more commonly in patients with high-risk alleles, suggesting an inherited predisposition. Most cases were found to have either the DR4 or DR3 allele. High-risk haplotypes included DR4-DQ8, DR3-DQ2, or DR4-DQ4 and were seen in 69% of cases.[3] The presence of islet antibodies before exposure to immunotherapy may also be a risk factor and needs further examination.

The incidence of autoimmune diabetes due to immunotherapy with checkpoint inhibitors has been found to be about 0.9%.[1] Ketoacidosis is the most common presentation and was seen in up to 75% of documented cases. Some cases also had evidence of pancreatitis. The time from initial exposure to presentation can be highly variable. The median length of time from initiation appears to depend on the ICI used. Using anti–PD-1/PD-L1 inhibitors, diabetes erupts after 4.5 cycles and earlier, and after only 2.7 cycles if used in combination with CTLA-4 inhibitors, as in this case. Although patients showed severe hyperglycemia with blood glucose levels over 1,000 mg/dL, the average

HbA$_{1c}$ at diagnosis was only 7.6–8%, indicating a rapid destruction of β-cells leading to acute insulin deficiency.[4] Low or undetectable C-peptide and insulin levels are usually observed. In about half of cases, islet cell antibodies are found, predominantly anti-GAD65. In this case, we cannot be sure that GAD antibodies did not exist before ICI therapy, as with other cases in the literature. The rarity of this phenomenon has discouraged routine antibody screening in all patients receiving ICIs. For this reason, presentation with ketoacidosis after combination therapy with PD-1/PD-L1 and CTLA-4 inhibitors as part of a rapid onset of autoimmune diabetes is the most typical presentation. Lipase levels are elevated in some patients.[5] Preexisting type 2 diabetes may confound the presentation and delay diagnosis. An abrupt worsening of glycemic control after exposure to ICIs should prompt careful glucose and ketone monitoring, and further evaluation with measurement of C-peptide and islet antibodies.

Given the severe insulin deficiency at presentation, these patients are invariably dependent on insulin for life. Use of advanced diabetes technology including insulin pumps and continuous glucose monitoring systems may prove invaluable in these cases.

COMMENTARY

With the increasing use of ICIs in the treatment of a variety of advanced malignancies, there is also an increasing awareness of the associated endocrinopathies that occur with these agents. The risk is even higher when these agents are used in combination to target different components of immune regulation. Of the reported endocrinopathies, adrenal insufficiency is considered the most critical due in part to increased risk for a life-threatening adrenal crisis. The patient presented in this case emphasizes that rapid onset of type 1 diabetes presenting as diabetic ketoacidosis can be as life-threatening as an adrenal crisis for some patients. Patients who develop ICI-associated endocrinopathies may present with nonspecific symptoms such as fatigue, weakness, nausea, visual impairments, or increased frequency of urination. A high index of suspicion is required to prompt endocrine evaluation that includes not only measurements of cortisol and thyroid function, but also electrolytes and blood glucose. Patient education regarding symptoms of concern early in the course of these therapies may allow earlier presentation before an acute crisis was observed in this patient.

Mary Korytkowski, MD

REFERENCES

1. Stamatouli AM, Quandt Z, Perdigoto AL, et al. Collateral damage: insulin-dependent diabetes induced with checkpoint inhibitors. *Diabetes* 2018;67: 1471–1480. https://doi.org/10.2337/dbi18-0002

2. Guleria I, Gubbels Bupp M, Dada S, et al. Mechanisms of PDL1-mediated regulation of autoimmune diabetes. *Clin Immunol* 2007;125:16–25. doi: 10.1016/j.clim.2007.05.013

3. Quandt Z, Young A, Anderson M. Immune checkpoint inhibitor diabetes mellitus: a novel form of autoimmune diabetes. *Clin Exp Immunol* 2020;200: 131–140. doi: 10.1111/cei.13424

4. Girotra M, Hansen A, Farooki A, et al. The current understanding of the endocrine effects from immune checkpoint inhibitors and recommendations for management. *JNCI Cancer Spectr* 2018;2:pky021. doi:10.1093/jncics/pky021

5. Gaudy C, Clévy C, Monestier S, et al. Anti-PD1 pembrolizumab can induce exceptional fulminant type 1 diabetes. *Diabetes Care* 2015;38:e182–e183. doi: 10.2337/dc15-1331

Case 14

Euglycemic Ketoacidosis in the Setting of COVID-19 Infection and Sodium–Glucose Cotransporter 2 Inhibitor Use

Olga Duchon, MD,[1] and Celeste Thomas, MD[1]

A 26-year-old man with a 3-year history of type 2 diabetes was admitted to the hospital with respiratory illness and abdominal symptoms attributed to coronavirus disease 2019 (COVID-19) infection. He had a history of intermittent insulin use and three or four hospital admissions for diabetic ketoacidosis (DKA) within the first 2 years of diagnosis. In the 3 months before this admission, he again discontinued insulin therapy but continued the sodium–glucose cotransporter 2 (SGLT2) inhibitor canagliflozin and glipizide that was prescribed by his primary care provider.

On admission, his glucose was 230 mg/dL, anion gap (AG) was 18, bicarbonate was 22 mEq/L, and venous pH was 7.39. A β-hydroxybutyrate level (ketones) was measured at 0.66 mmol/L (reference range <0.3 mmol/L). Over the next several hours, the β-hydroxybutyrate increased to 2.79 mmol/L with an associated AG of 21 and decrease in bicarbonate to 18 mEq/L with a blood glucose of 208 mg/dL. He was transferred to the intensive care unit (ICU) for intensified management of his DKA. Canagliflozin was stopped upon admission.

After nearly 24 h of insulin infusion at an average rate of 7 units/h in combination with dextrose-containing intravenous (IV) fluids, he was transitioned to subcutaneous insulin therapy and weaned off the IV insulin infusion. Despite some improvement in his presenting symptoms, his oral intake remained poor. Three days after discontinuation of the IV insulin infusion, he experienced worsening abdominal complaints. His β-hydroxybutyrate was elevated with a widening AG despite blood glucose levels remaining in the low 200s. It was recommended that the patient be treated for DKA with an IV insulin infusion, which is restricted to the ICU at this institution. Because of limited bed availability, transfer to the ICU was not possible. Furthermore, because of this patient's active COVID-19 status, his DKA treatment consisted of point-of-care blood glucose checks and subcutaneous insulin administration every 4 h, with maximum frequency of blood draws every 12 h.

Application of protocols identified in the literature for treating DKA with subcutaneous insulin proved impractical because of the limited availability

[1]Endocrinology, University of Chicago Medicine, Chicago, Illinois.

DOI: 10.2337/9781580407663.14

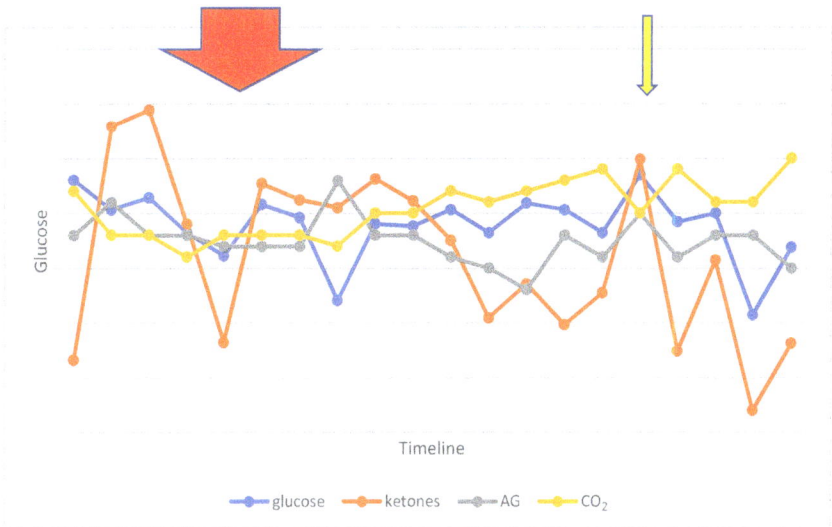

Figure 14.1—Trends in selected components of the metabolic profile. Glucose is in mg/dL; β-hydroxybutyrate is in mmol/L × 100; AG × 10; CO_2 mEq/L × 10. Red arrow = insulin infusion; yellow arrow = subcutaneous treatment initiated.

of nursing personnel and inability to administer high volumes of fluids. For these reasons, the patient was started on 5% dextrose at 60 cc/h with administration of subcutaneous insulin lispro 0.05 units/kg every 4 h. His dose of basal insulin glargine was increased to 0.25 units/kg. This patient ultimately received ~0.07 units/kg insulin lispro every 4 h, with eventual clinical and metabolic recovery. A carbohydrate-consistent diet was initiated, and he was transitioned off of IV dextrose. Figure 14.1 shows the trends.

Euglycemic diabetic ketoacidosis (eDKA) is a rare but known complication of treatment with SGLT2 inhibitors. SGLT2 inhibitors are a relatively new class of medications for treating type 2 diabetes that are gaining increasing use in light of demonstrated improved cardiovascular and renal outcomes. Side effects, such as eDKA, remain a concern, and more information is needed regarding possible triggers and the eDKA timeline to inform guidelines and promote vigilance among prescribers.

DKA is a decompensated metabolic state associated with pathologically high serum and urine concentrations of ketone bodies that result from unregulated lipolysis with release of free fatty acids, which undergo β-oxidation to provide a backup source of energy for tissues. The diagnostic criteria for euglycemic DKA are the same as for DKA (bicarbonate <18, pH <7.3, and ketonemia); however, blood glucose levels are usually lower than levels typically associated with DKA and are often below 200 mg/dL.

The precipitants for eDKA that were identified in the case and are most commonly described include the use of the long-acting SGLT2 inhibitor canagliflozin, decreased oral intake (e.g., starvation), stress, cessation or decrease in exogenous insulin, and infection. Other identified precipitants include surgery, strenuous exercise, and pregnancy.

SGLT2 inhibitors were first implicated in the pathogenesis of eDKA in 2014.[1] The incidence of DKA in patients with type 1 diabetes treated with SGLT2 inhibitors is reported to be as high as 9.4%, while the incidence is 0.2% with type 2 diabetes. The mechanism of eDKA development while on SGLT2 inhibitors resembles that of "starvation ketosis."[2,3] The main driver of the metabolic deterioration is thought to be increased glucosuria and increased glucose utilization by tissues due to increased insulin sensitivity, ultimately leading to decreased serum glucose, decreased insulin production, and both direct and indirect stimulation of glucagon secretion. A decrease in the insulin-to-glucagon ratio has been long known to be the main driver of switch from glucose to fat metabolism. Inhibition of SGLT2 also increases $Na+$ excretion that leads to increased ketone reabsorption. Another possible mechanism is an increased synthesis of fibroblast growth factor 21 (FGF21) by adipocytes that play a role in the adaptation to metabolic states requiring increased fatty acid oxidation such as fasting.

In the case of COVID-19 infection, anorexia and anosmia likely contribute to decreased carbohydrate consumption, tilting the balance towards ketogenesis and starvation ketosis. This patient also had more than one previous hospitalization for DKA, suggesting the presence of relative insulin deficiency that was further exacerbated by acute illness. The treatment of eDKA is essentially the same as hyperglycemic DKA with the exception of earlier introduction of dextrose-containing fluids. Given concerns about excess fluid resuscitation in the presence of active COVID-19 infection and efforts to reduce workforce exposure, the empiric approach described above was used on a general medicine ward and proved effective in this case.

COMMENTARY

The patient presented in this case description likely had either type 1 diabetes with residual insulin secretion or ketosis-prone type 2 diabetes that put him at higher risk for developing eDKA given the preexisting insulin deficiency. His noncompliance with previously prescribed insulin therapy further contributed to his risk for eDKA while receiving the long-acting SGLT2 inhibitor canagliflozin, which likely contributed to the recurrence of eDKA several days after resolution of the original event. SGLT2 inhibitors should be discontinued 72 h before planned surgical procedures where patients may be in the fasting state for prolonged periods. These agents should also be discontinued at the time of hospital admission for patients with COVID-19 infection to minimize risk for metabolic deterioration.

This case also illustrates the reality of providing the complex care these patients require when admitted to the hospital. An established DKA treatment protocol was implemented at his initial presentation, but because of an overwhelmed health care setting later in his hospitalization, he was treated with a modified protocol. The authors successfully treated this patient's recurrent DKA with modified administration of IV fluids and subcutaneous basal-bolus insulin therapy, emphasizing the important issues of fluid resuscitation, electrolyte replacement, and monitored insulin therapy to resolve this potentially life-threatening complication.

Mary Korytkowski, MD

REFERENCES

1. Ogawa W. Euglycemic diabetic ketoacidosis induced by SGLT2 inhibitors: possible mechanism and contributing factors. *J Diabetes Investig* 2016;7: 135–138

2. Grey NJ. Physiologic mechanisms in the development of starvation ketosis in man. *Diabetes* 1975;24:10–16

3. Yu X. Newer perspectives of mechanisms for euglycemic diabetic ketoacidosis. *Int J Endocrinol* 2018;2018:7074868

Case 15

Euglycemic Diabetic Ketoacidosis Due to Sodium–Glucose Cotransporter 2 Inhibitor Use

Diana Soliman, MD,[1] and Nicole Jelesoff, MD[1]

A 79-year-old male with type 2 diabetes diagnosed at age 49 years presented with worsening generalized weakness, subacute functional decline, nausea, vomiting, diarrhea, and decreased oral intake. He had a history of regionally advanced melanoma and hypophysitis with development of secondary adrenal insufficiency and hypothyroidism related to treatment with ipilimumab and nivolumab.

Before admission, his antihyperglycemic agents were glipizide 5 mg, metformin 1,000 mg twice daily, and empagliflozin 25 mg daily. Empagliflozin was added to his regimen 1 year before admission. His HbA_{1c} was 8% at time of hospital admission.

On presentation, his serum bicarbonate was 18 mEq/L, anion gap was 14, and serum χ-hydroxybutyrate was 1.05 mmol/L. His glucose was 185 mg/dL, and urinalysis was significant for 3+ glucose and 1+ ketones, all consistent with a diagnosis of euglycemic diabetic ketoacidosis (eDKA). His renal function was normal. His oral antihyperglycemic medications were held and intravenous (IV) fluids were initiated together with an IV insulin drip (Table 15.1).

On day 2 of admission, his serum χ-hydroxybutyrate rose to 2.39 mmol/L. On day 3, his urine ketones were negative, and the insulin drip was stopped. On day 4, his serum χ-hydroxybutyrate rose to 1.34 mmol/L with a serum bicarbonate of 18 mEq/L and an anion gap of 11. At this point, the insulin drip was restarted. On day 6, when his serum ketones were negative, the insulin drip was stopped again. On day 7, his serum χ-hydroxybutyrate was slightly elevated to 0.47 mmol/L without an increase in his anion gap. During his admission, his diet was restricted to 60 g carbohydrates per meal. On day 7, his dietary intake of carbohydrates was liberalized, and his serum ketones became negative shortly thereafter. Glucosuria persisted for several days after empagliflozin was stopped, even in the setting of near-normal blood glucose levels. By day 8, the glucosuria had resolved.

There was concern for immunotherapy-induced type 1 diabetes; however, his GAD antibodies were negative, and a postprandial C-peptide was

[1]Duke University Division of Endocrinology, Diabetes and Metabolism, Duke University School of Medicine, Durham, North Carolina.

DOI: 10.2337/9781580407663.15

Table 15.1—Patient's lab values during hospitalization

	Day 1	Day 2	Day 3	Day 4	Day 5	Day 6	Day 7	Day 8
Serum bicarbonate (mEq/L)	18	17	23	18	17	20	23	24
Serum anion gap	14	15	7	11	11	8	6	7
Serum glucose (mg/dL)	185	194	136	128	160	123	86	140
Serum χ-hydroxy-butyrate (mmol/L)	1.05	2.39	—	1.34	1.87	<0.18	0.47	<0.18
Urine glucose	3+	—	3+	3+	3+	2+	3+	Negative
Urine ketones	1+	—	Negative	1+	Negative	Negative	Negative	Negative
Notes	Insulin drip started		Insulin drip stopped	Insulin drip restarted		Insulin drip stopped	Carbohy-drate intake lib-eralized	

Dashes indicate not checked.

detectable at 1.2 nmol/L. His presentation was consistent with eDKA due to empagliflozin use.

eDKA secondary to sodium–glucose cotransporter 2 (SGLT2) inhibitor use was recently described in the literature. It is important to remind patients to stop SGLT2 inhibitors in the setting of decreased oral intake, vomiting, prolonged fasting, and acute illness. It is also recommended that patients stop SGLT2 inhibitors 72 h before any elective surgery/procedure or planned strenuous physical activity, such as running a marathon.[1] This case illustrates that eDKA caused by SGLT2 inhibitors can be prolonged, and serum ketones are preferred to urine ketones for monitoring.

SGLT2 inhibitors work to lower blood glucose levels by preventing the reabsorption of glucose at the proximal convoluted renal tubules. Several mechanisms are proposed to explain the development of eDKA in patients receiving these agents. Insulin deficiency and glucagon excess play a central role in the development of DKA. By increasing urinary glucose excretion, SGLT2 inhibitors lower blood glucose, which leads to a reduction in insulin secretion.[2] The relative insulin deficiency leads to an increase in lipolysis resulting in increased production of free fatty acids, which are subsequently converted to ketones in the liver. Excess glucagon occurs because of 1) feedback from insulin deficiency and 2) a direct effect of SGLT2 inhibitors on pancreatic α-cells.[2] Because serum glucose remains in the near-normal range in eDKA, there can often be delays in diagnosis and therapeutic intervention.

The pharmacological half-life of empagliflozin is about 13 h, so the drug should be eliminated within 3 days.[1] In this case, our patient continued to have glucosuria for several days after the medication was stopped, even though his blood glucose levels were only mildly elevated, suggesting that the drug's biologic effect persists for longer than expected. There have been similar reports of patients with prolonged glucosuria after cessation of SGLT2 inhibitors.[3]

In the case presented, the insulin drip was stopped when his anion gap metabolic acidosis resolved and *urine* ketones became negative. Shortly thereafter, his *serum* ketones were again found to be positive. It is recommended that serum ketones be used to diagnose and monitor eDKA secondary to SGLT2 inhibitors, since these agents can decrease urinary excretion of ketone bodies.[1,2] However, a recent study found that elevated β-hydroxybutyrate levels in these patients are related more to overproduction than to reduced renal clearance.[4] The three ketone bodies that accumulate in DKA are acetoacetic acid, β-hydroxybutyric acid, and acetone. The dominant ketone body in ketoacidosis and the one predominantly excreted in the urine is β-hydroxybutyrate. This finding has important clinical implications when using urine ketone test strips, since these detect acetoacetate and not β-hydroxybutyrate, meaning that ketonuria may potentially be missed.

Caution is recommended when placing patients treated with SGLT2 inhibitors on carbohydrate-restricted diets, as occurred with this patient. Together with his decreased oral intake, the low-carbohydrate diet may have contributed to prolonged ketosis. After the insulin drip was stopped the second time, his serum ketones were again mildly elevated. After liberalization of his diet to include more carbohydrates, the ketosis resolved. As ketogenic diets gain popularity, providers should keep in mind that these low-carbohydrate diets may potentially trigger eDKA in patients on SGLT2 inhibitors.

In conclusion, this case illustrates the challenges associated with treating eDKA due to SGLT2 inhibitor use. It is vital to counsel patients when to temporarily stop SGLT2 inhibitors to minimize the risk of eDKA. Providers should keep in mind that eDKA secondary to SGLT2 inhibitor use may have a longer course than expected. The measurement of serum ketones, specifically β-hydroxybutyrate, and monitoring of urine glucose may be necessary and preferred over using the serum anion gap and urine ketone monitoring to document effective resolution of SGLT2 inhibitor–induced ketoacidosis.

COMMENTARY

This case represents a patient with a prolonged episode of eDKA related to use of an SGLT2 inhibitor in the setting of an acute illness with reduced oral intake. There is a need to educate patients to discontinue these medications in the event of an acute illness associated with reductions in oral intake. Further restricting carbohydrate intake as his gastrointestinal symptoms resolved contributed to the recurrence of DKA, although it is not clear if insulin therapy was continued after discontinuation of the IV insulin infusion. The recommendation has been made that patients treated with SGLT2 inhibitors be provided with urine ketone test strips in the event of an acute illness. This patient illustrates that negative urine ketones cannot definitively eliminate the possibility that a patient has developed eDKA and that laboratory testing with a metabolic panel may be necessary for many patients who report symptoms, as described in this case. Finally, it is of interest that this patient was receiving therapy with a combination of immune checkpoint inhibitors that have been demonstrated to cause autoimmune-mediated diabetes with an ongoing insulin requirement, for which measurement of GAD antibodies was indicated. Taken altogether, this patient represents the complexity of management and decision-making needed for the successful outcome of these patients with multiple risk factors for development of DKA.

Mary Korytkowski, MD

REFERENCES

1. Handelsman Y, Henry RR, Bloomgarden ZT, et al. American Association of Clinical Endocrinologists and American College of Endocrinology position statement on the association of SGLT-2 inhibitors on diabetic ketoacidosis. *Endocr Pract* 2016;22:753–762. doi:10.4158/EP161292.PS

2. Taylor SI, Blaummm JE, Rother KI. SGLT2 inhibitors may predispose to ketoacidosis. *J Clin Endocrinol Metab* 2015;100:2849–2852. doi:10.1210/jc.2015-1884

3. Alhassan S, Rudoni M, Alfonso-Jaume MA, Jaume JC. Protracted glycosuria after discontinuation of sodium-glucose cotransporter 2 inhibitors: implications for weekly dosing and extended risk of euglycemic diabetes ketoacidosis. *J Diabetes* 2019;11:410–411. doi:10.1111/1753-0407.12885

4. Ferrannini E, Baldi S, Frascerra S, et al. Renal handling of ketones in response to sodium–glucose cotransporter 2 inhibition in patients with type 2 diabetes. *Diabetes Care* 2017;40:771–776. doi:10.2337/dc16-2724

Case 16

A Case of Euglycemic Diabetic Ketoacidosis After Initiation of Ketogenic Diet in a Patient With Type 2 Diabetes on a Sodium–Glucose Cotransporter 2 (SGLT2) Inhibitor

Matthew P. Gilbert, DO, MPH,[1] and Amy Shah, DO[1]

A 52-year-old Caucasian female with a past medical history of well-controlled type 2 diabetes, hypertension, and dyslipidemia presented to the emergency department with a 3-day history of severe headache associated with nausea, neck pain, and photophobia. Her outpatient diabetes regimen consisted of metformin 1,000 mg twice a day, linagliptin (a dipeptidyl peptidase-4 [DPP-4] inhibitor) 5 mg daily, and empagliflozin (a sodium–glucose cotransporter 2 [SGLT2] inhibitor) 25 mg daily. She reported starting a ketogenic diet 4 months before admission with an objective 17-lb weight loss after she had prior success with extremely low-carbohydrate/ketogenic diets in the past. Imaging on admission revealed a nontraumatic subarachnoid hemorrhage. Initial laboratory evaluation in the emergency department included a venous pH of 7.2, bicarbonate levels of 13 mmol/L, an anion gap of 23 mEq/L, elevated χ-hydroxybutyrate of 7.2 mmol/L, and >3.0 mmol/L ketones in her urine. Her serum glucose at time of presentation was 125 mEq/L with an HbA_{1c} of 6.1%. Endocrinology was consulted and the patient was diagnosed with euglycemic diabetic ketoacidosis (eDKA). She was placed briefly on an insulin drip with resulting rapid resolution of her DKA. At discharge, she was instructed to continue her previous doses of metformin and DPP-4 inhibitor. Basaglar (a long-acting insulin) was added at 18 units (0.2 units/kg), but it was eventually tapered and subsequently discontinued. The patient's SGLT2 inhibitor was discontinued at discharge and she was instructed to also discontinue her ketogenic diet. The patient has been doing well clinically since being discharged from the hospital. She continues with excellent control of her type 2 diabetes using a combination of metformin and linagliptin (a DPP-4 inhibitor) in conjunction with an improved diet and regular exercise.

SGLT2 inhibitors are a class of antihyperglycemic agents that inhibit glucose reuptake in the kidney. Whether used as monotherapy or in combination with other antihyperglycemic therapies, SGLT2 inhibitors have been

[1]Department of Medicine, Division of Endocrinology and Diabetes, Larner College of Medicine at The University of Vermont, Burlington, Vermont.

DOI: 10.2337/9781580407663.16

associated with a risk of eDKA.[1] The condition of eDKA was originally defined as DKA with plasma sodium glucose levels <300 mg/dL, and it is typically reported in young female patients with type 1 diabetes.[2] The primary cause of eDKA is reduced availability of carbohydrate in conjunction with reduced insulin doses.[2] The eDKA reported in patients with type 2 diabetes treated with SGLT2 inhibitors, however, has a different mechanism— the lowering of blood glucose by SGLT2 inhibitors results in decreased insulin secretion and an increase in counter-regulatory hormones such as epinephrine, cortisol, and glucagon.[2] There is also evidence that SGLT2 inhibitors can directly induce glucagon release. The subsequent decreased insulin-to-glucagon ratio causes an increase in lipolysis with increased circulating free fatty acids and ketogenesis.[2]

For patients with type 2 diabetes or prediabetes, low-carbohydrate diets have shown a potential to improve glycemic control and lipid profiles.[3] Unfortunately, there remains significant variation in the definition of a "low-carbohydrate diet" within the clinical literature. Therefore, interpretation of this literature concerning potential benefits in patients with type 2 diabetes has remained challenging. It is recommended that clinicians regularly review individualized meal-planning guidance with patients interested in low-carbohydrate diets.[3] The American Diabetes Association recommends that certain patient groups may not be appropriate for low-carbohydrate diets. These groups include patients using SGLT2 inhibitors because of the potential risk of eDKA.[3] Even in patients with sufficient insulin secretory capacity, a combination of strict adherence to a low-carbohydrate diet combined with treatment with a SGLT2 inhibitor may precipitate eDKA. Ketosis results from the restriction of carbohydrate usage for energy production offset by an increased reliance on fat oxidation to meet energy requirements.[2] Yabe et al.[4] suggested, in a randomized, exploratory study of Japanese individuals with type 2 diabetes treated with a SGLT2 inhibitor, that the carbohydrate content of meals can play an important role in SGLT2 inhibitor–associated hepatic ketogenesis and onset of eDKA. This clinical trial showed that patients receiving a carbohydrate-restricted diet (177 g carbohydrates per day) showed increased ketosis compared to the group receiving 244 g carbohydrates per day.[4] We believe that the combination of an acute clinical event (subarachnoid hemorrhage), treatment with a SGLT2 inhibitor, and a ketogenic diet contributed to our patient's presentation with eDKA.

In the first case series of eDKA associated with use of SGLT2 inhibitors, Peters et al.[5] reported that, at the time of initial presentation, acute care providers often failed to recognize the clinical signs and symptoms of eDKA, leading to unnecessary testing and treatment. The delay in recognition of this serious complication of diabetes is often due to the lack of significant hyperglycemia usually associated with DKA in patients treated with SGLT2 inhibitors. In our case, the patient presented with headache and a subsequent discovery of a subarachnoid hemorrhage. The physician in the emergency department was aware of the possibility of eDKA given her treatment with an SGLT2 inhibitor and promptly recognized her low bicarbonate and nausea as potential signs of eDKA. We believe the early recognition of possible eDKA led to immediate and appropriate treatment, thus contributing to her quick recovery. This case illustrates the clinical pearl that patients with type 2 diabetes who present with nausea, vomiting, shortness of breath, or fatigue in the setting of SGLT2 inhibitor therapy should be evaluated for diabetic ketoacidosis even in the setting of normal or near-normal blood glucose levels.

The clinical presentation of patients with eDKA is similar to that of patients with hyperglycemic DKA. Patients with eDKA can present with nausea, vomiting, shortness of breath, generalized malaise, lethargy, loss of appetite, fatigue, and/or abdominal pain. The initial laboratory evaluation for eDKA is similar to that for patients with DKA. As with our patient's experience, most patients with eDKA recover quickly after prompt recognition and appropriate treatment via established DKA protocols.

The available clinical evidence has shown that SGLT2 inhibitor–associated eDKA is rare, and it is triggered by known precipitants such as acute illness, major surgical procedures, dehydration, or initiation of extremely low-carbohydrate/ketogenic diets.[1] Therefore, eDKA can be prevented by withholding SGLT2 inhibitors when indicated, counseling patients about sick-day management, and recommending against extremely low-carbohydrate or ketogenic diets in patients treated with SGLT2 inhibitors.

COMMENTARY

Current recommendations advise against use of SGLT2 inhibitors in patients with type 1 diabetes or ketosis-prone type 2 diabetes given the higher risk for developing eDKA. Prolonged periods of fasting and use of increasingly popular ketogenic diets are described as potential factors that can increase the risk of eDKA in patients with type 2 diabetes treated with these agents. The patient in this case had well-controlled type 2 diabetes and was following a normal diet preceding her acute presentation with a subarachnoid hemorrhage and eDKA. This result suggests that any patient treated with these agents can be at risk for the occurrence of this potentially life-threatening complication. Prompt identification and treatment of this complication by emergency department personnel resulted in rapid resolution of her DKA with eventual return to well-controlled type 2 diabetes with noninsulin therapy. This case emphasizes recommendations that serum ketones be measured in any patient presenting with symptoms of nausea, vomiting, or malaise while taking SGLT2 inhibitors. Providing patients with test strips and instructions for urine ketone testing at home could facilitate early diagnosis and treatment for patients at home who experience these symptoms.

Mary Korytkowski, MD

REFERENCES

1. Goldenberg RM, Berard LD, Cheng AYY, et al. SGLT2 inhibitor-associated diabetic ketoacidosis: clinical review and recommendations for prevention and diagnosis. *Clin Ther* 2016;38:2654–2664

2. Rosenstock J, Ferrannini E. Euglycemic diabetic ketoacidosis: a predictable, detectable, and preventable safety concern with SGLT2 inhibitors. *Diabetes Care* 2015;38:1638–1642

3. American Diabetes Association. 5. Facilitating behavior change and well-being to improve health outcomes: *Standards of Medical Care in Diabetes-2020. Diabetes Care* 2020;43(Suppl. 1):S48–S65

4. Yabe D, Iwasaki M, Kuwata H, et al. Sodium-glucose co-transporter-2 inhibitor use and dietary carbohydrate intake in Japanese individuals with type 2 diabetes: a randomized, open-label, 3-arm parallel comparative, exploratory study. *Diabetes Obes Metab* 2017;19:739–743

5. Peters AL, Buschur EO, Buse JB, Cohan P, Diner JC, Hirsch IB. Euglycemic diabetic ketoacidosis: a potential complication of treatment with sodium-glucose cotransporter 2 inhibition. *Diabetes Care* 2015;38:1687–1693

Case 17

Diabetic Ketoacidosis in End-Stage Renal Disease: A Unique Challenge

VISHNU GARLA, MD,[1,2] ANGELA SUBAUSTE, MD,[2] AND LILLIAN F. LIEN, MD[2]

A 47-year-old female patient with type 1 diabetes, end-stage renal disease (ESRD), and congestive heart failure was admitted with chest pain and dyspnea. Physical examination was significant for bibasilar crepitation, jugular venous distention, and pedal edema consistent with volume overload. Laboratory assessment revealed hyperglycemia, hyponatremia, metabolic acidosis, and elevated blood urea nitrogen, creatinine, and brain natriuretic peptide (Table 17.1).

Electrocardiogram was not significant for ischemic changes. The chest radiograph showed bilateral pleural effusions. Furosemide and glargine insulin were started for the treatment of hypervolemia and hyperglycemia, respectively. Over the next 24 h, hyperglycemia and acidosis worsened significantly (Table 17.1). Serum χ-hydroxybutyrate was high at 82.49 (0.2–2.81 mg/dL). Endocrinology was consulted for the management of diabetic ketoacidosis (DKA). Intravenous (IV) insulin infusion was started at a lower dose than usual (0.5 units/h to be titrated up to a maximum of 2 units/h) as opposed to the conventional DKA algorithm (0.1 units/kg/h) to prevent recurrent hypoglycemia (as is common when higher rates are used in ESRD). A dextrose infusion (50–150 mL/h) was initiated to avoid hypoglycemia while allowing insulin to infuse. Over the next 48 h, the acidosis resolved, and the χ-hydroxybutyrate normalized (Table 17.1). The IV insulin infusion was discontinued and transitioned to a subcutaneous basal-bolus regimen.

DKA is a life-threatening hyperglycemic emergency. Management of DKA with concomitant ESRD is a unique challenge, since therapies for DKA (fluid resuscitation, IV insulin, and potassium replacement) are essential but potentially dangerous in ESRD.[1] ESRD patients with DKA are at a higher risk of complications than DKA patients with normal renal function. They have an increased risk of hypoglycemia, a higher need for mechanical ventilation, and a

[1]Department of Internal Medicine, Mississippi Center for Clinical and Translational Research (MCCTR), University of Mississippi Medical Center, Jackson, Mississippi.
[2]Division of Endocrinology, Metabolism, and Diabetes, University of Mississippi Medical Center, Jackson, Mississippi.

   DOI: 10.2337/9781580407663.17

Table 17.1—Laboratory assessment

	Baseline	24 h	48 h
Serum glucose (74–106 mg/dL)	448	169	131
Serum sodium (136–145 mmol/L)	131	135	133
Serum potassium (3.5–4.5 mmol/L)	5.3	3.5	3.5
Serum bicarbonate (22–29 mmol/L)	6	18	20
Serum chloride (98–107 mmol/L)	88	95	96
Anion gap (6–14 mmol/L)	37	22	17
Blood urea nitrogen (6–20 mg/dL)	61	59	51
Serum creatinine (0.51–0.95 mg/dL)	8.02	7.99	7.62
Serum phosphorous (2.7–4.5 mg/dL)	7	6.9	
β-Hydroxybutyrate (0.2–2.81 mg/dL)	82.49	31.69	0.61
proBNP (5–125 pg/mL)	40,476		

proBNP, pro brain natriuretic peptide.

longer length of stay in the hospital. Despite the increased risk, there are no specific guidelines for the management of DKA in ESRD.[2]

DKA is characterized by hyperglycemia (blood glucose >250 mg/dL, with the exception of euglycemic DKA), metabolic acidosis (serum bicarbonate <18 mEq/L), and ketonemia. The underlying defects in DKA are insulin deficiency and an increase in levels of counter-regulatory hormones. These defects lead to decreased glucose utilization and increased lipolysis and free fatty acid formation. The free fatty acids are converted to ketones. The use of ketones for energy production overwhelms normal buffering capacity, resulting in metabolic acidosis. Hyperglycemia results in increased tonicity and osmotic diuresis, which may result in hypovolemia. Insulin deficiency causes a transcellular shift of potassium and phosphorous to the extracellular fluid.[3]

In ESRD, the above-mentioned pathophysiological changes take a different course. ESRD patients with DKA are at increased risk of hypoglycemia due to decreased renal gluconeogenesis as well as insulin retention. In DKA with preserved renal function, acid excretion increases substantially, attenuating the metabolic acidosis. However, in the presence of ESRD, metabolic acidosis develops rapidly because of the kidneys' inability to excrete acid. Pulmonary edema due to volume overload may impede the development of respiratory alkalosis as a compensatory mechanism for the metabolic acidosis. Hyperglycemia can lead to extracellular fluid expansion, as mentioned above; however, because of the lack of renal function in ESRD, this excess fluid cannot be eliminated, resulting in hypervolemia. This result is in contrast to DKA with preserved renal function in which hypovolemia is the primary concern. Insulin induces hypokalemia and hypophosphatemia by promoting the intracellular shift of potassium and phosphorous. ESRD is associated with hyperkalemia and hyperphosphatemia due to decreased renal clearance. Insulin deficiency can potentially worsen hyperkalemia and hyperphosphatemia.[1,2]

Diagnosing DKA in ESRD patients is a challenge due to persistent metabolic acidosis often observed in these patients and alteration of bicarbonate levels secondary to oral supplementation or dialysis. Worsening metabolic acidosis or persistence despite hemodialysis could indicate the development of DKA. The lack of glycogen stores and renal gluconeogenesis may result in milder hyperglycemia, further confounding diagnosis. Assessing β-hydroxybutyrate level is useful for establishing the diagnosis and monitoring of DKA in ESRD patients.[2,4]

The cornerstones for the treatment of DKA are insulin therapy, along with fluid and electrolyte management. Because patients with ESRD and DKA are prone to hypoglycemia; it is recommended to start insulin infusion at a lower rate compared to non-ESRD patients with DKA. Seddik et al.[1] recommended a starting insulin infusion rate of 0.05–0.07 units/kg/h titrated to decrease glucose by 50–75 mg/dL hourly. Patients with type 1 diabetes and ESRD are the most prone to hypoglycemia. In these patients, we recommend maintaining an insulin infusion rate at a minimum of 0.5 and a maximum of 3 units/h. As above, the IV insulin infusion rate is titrated hourly, to decrease blood glucose by 50–75 mg/dL hourly. Furthermore, simultaneous insulin and dextrose infusions may be necessary to inhibit ketogenesis and avoid hypoglycemia.[1,5]

In DKA with preserved renal function, aggressive fluid replacement is necessary to aid in renal ketone clearance. However, given that patients in DKA with ESRD are prone to hypervolemia, fluid replacement should be conservative and given through small boluses (250–500 mL).[1] Unlike DKA with normal renal function, DKA with ESRD is associated with increased total body potassium; therefore, routine supplementation of potassium is not recommended. Hypokalemia is treated with potassium chloride to a target of 3.5 mmol/L. ESRD is also associated with phosphorous retention, and replacement is recommended only for hypophosphatemia of <1.5 mg/dL.[5]

The role of hemodialysis to correct the electrolyte abnormalities of DKA has not been well studied. Emergency dialysis can be considered for severe hyperkalemia with electrocardiogram (ECG) manifestations, profound acidosis, and pulmonary edema. Continuous renal replacement therapy is better suited for patients with hemodynamic instability.[1]

In conclusion, DKA with ESRD differs from conventional DKA in significant ways (Table 17.2). Rather than focusing on serum bicarbonate, the diagnosis of DKA in ESRD is made by assessing β-hydroxybutyrate in a patient with persistent or worsening acidosis. The management of DKA in ESRD includes conservative administration of fluids and insulin to simultaneously inhibit ketogenesis and prevent hypoglycemia. Routine replacement of potassium and phosphorous is not recommended. Emergent dialysis is indicated for the management of profound acidosis, hyperkalemia with ECG changes, and pulmonary edema. Further studies are needed for the development of specific guidelines for the management of DKA in ESRD.

Table 17.2—Recommendations for management of DKA in patients with ESRD and type 1 diabetes

Insulin therapy • Continuously infuse insulin with conservative rates, ranging from 0.5 to 3 units/h. Goal is to lower blood glucose by 50–75 mg/dL hourly. • Monitor β-hydroxybutyrate levels to assess for resolution of ketogenesis. • Dextrose infusions can be used to avoid hypoglycemia and permit continued insulin infusion to suppress ketogenesis.
Fluid and electrolyte management • Conservative fluid management (250- to 500-mL boluses) is recommended to avoid hypervolemia. • Closely monitor cardiac and hemodynamic status. • Routine supplementation of potassium and phosphorous is not recommended. • Hypokalemia (<3.5 mmol/L) can be treated with potassium chloride supplementation. • Hypophosphatemia (<1.5 mmol/L) can be treated with IV supplementation.
Indications for dialysis • Profound metabolic acidosis • Severe hyperkalemia with ECG manifestations • Severe pulmonary edema

COMMENTARY

The occurrence of DKA in patients with diabetes and ESRD can be difficult to both identify and treat. The degree of metabolic acidosis observed in this patient at presentation prompted measurement of β-hydroxybutyrate level that was markedly elevated and confirmed the contribution of DKA to this patient's acute presentation. The majority of published and hospital-based protocols for DKA management specifically exclude patients with ESRD, with the caveat that these patients require individualized therapy with cautious fluid replacement and insulin therapy to avoid hypervolemia and hypoglycemia, as well as electrolyte abnormalities. However, there is little available guidance for these patients beyond these general principles. This case illustrates successful resolution of DKA with low-dose IV insulin therapy and cautious fluid replacement with dextrose-containing solutions. Table 17.2 provides a summary approach that can be useful to others in the management of these patients.

Mary Korytkowski, MD

REFERENCES

1. Seddik AA, Bashier A, Alhadari AK, et al. Challenges in management of diabetic ketoacidosis in hemodialysis patients, case presentation and review of literature. *Diabetes Metab Syndr* 2019;13:2481–2487

2. Galindo RJ, Pasquel FJ, Fayfman M, et al. Clinical characteristics and outcomes of patients with end-stage renal disease hospitalized with diabetes ketoacidosis. *BMJ Open Diabetes Res Care* 2020;8:e000763

3. Maletkovic J, Drexler A. Diabetic ketoacidosis and hyperglycemic hyperosmolar state. *Endocrinol Metab Clin North Am* 2013;42:677–695

4. Sheikh-Ali M, Karon BS, Basu A, et al. Can serum beta-hydroxybutyrate be used to diagnose diabetic ketoacidosis? *Diabetes Care* 2008;31:643–647

5. Varma R, Karim M. Lesson of the month 1: diabetic ketoacidosis in established renal failure. *Clin Med (Lond)* 2016;16:392–393

Case 18

Euglycemic Diabetic Ketoacidosis in a Patient With Type 1 Diabetes Treated With a Sodium–Glucose Cotransporter 2 (SGLT2) Inhibitor While on a Ketogenic Diet

Jessica Castellanos-Diaz, MD,[1,2] Julio Leey-Casella, MD,[1,2] Kenneth Cusi, MD,[1,2] and Sushma Kadiyala, MD[1,2]

A 70-year-old female with unspecified diabetes presented to the emergency department complaining of nausea, dizziness, and anorexia for 4 days. She was diagnosed with diabetes at age 37 years. In her record, both type 1 diabetes and type 2 diabetes were listed as diagnoses. No prior C-peptide or serum antibodies were available. She had peripheral neuropathy and early stage 3 chronic kidney disease without proteinuria. She had no known history of cardiovascular disease or any previous admissions for diabetic ketoacidosis (DKA). (Laboratory results summarized in Table 18.1).

The patient had transferred her care to a new provider for presumed type 2 diabetes with HbA$_{1c}$ of 9.0%. Despite her normal BMI of 21 kg/m^2 and age, she was started on a ketogenic diet (KD) to improve her glycemic status and lower her insulin requirements. Medications were changed from insulin only (glargine 20 units at bedtime and insulin aspart with meals) to glargine 20 units daily, metformin 1,000 mg twice a day, and empagliflozin 12.5 mg daily. A reason for this change was to improve the safety of her regimen and reduce the frequency of hypoglycemia, since reported home blood glucose readings of 50–60 mg/dL on several occasions were attributed primarily to the short-acting insulin. She had been on this regimen for 4 weeks, having lost approximately 12 lb (per chart review) before her presentation to the emergency department. Physical exam and vital signs were unremarkable, except for tachypnea.

She was diagnosed with euglycemic DKA (eDKA) and admitted to the hospital for management. The triggering factor was likely due to a combination of starvation, KD-induced acidosis, and empagliflozin. Other causes such as infection, pancreatitis, a cardiac event, drug use, or alcohol use were excluded. The patient was initially treated with intravenous (IV) normal saline, 0.9% 500-mL bolus, and subcutaneous insulin. Dietary intake was soon reinstated with the goal of restoring carbohydrate intake to reverse

[1]Department of Medicine, Division of Endocrinology, Diabetes and Metabolism, Malcom Randall Veteran Hospital, Gainesville, Florida. [2]Department of Medicine, Division of Endocrinology, Diabetes and Metabolism, University of Florida College of Medicine, Gainesville, Florida.

DOI: 10.2337/9781580407663.18

Table 18.1 — Initial labs at emergency department evaluation

Laboratory test (reference range)	Result
Serum glucose (65–100 mg/dL)	136 mg/dL
Carbon dioxide (20–30 mmol/L)	10 mmol/L
Anion gap (1–10 mEq/L)	27 mEq/L
Venous blood gas pH (7.35–7.45)	7.1
β-Hydroxybutyrate (0.02–0.27 mmol/L)	8.8 mmol/L
Urine glucose (0 mg/dL)	>500 mg/dL
Urine ketones (negative)	Moderate
Potassium (3.5–5.0 mmol/L)	4.1 mmol/L
Creatinine (0.84–1.21 mg/dL)	0.80 mg/dL

the deleterious effect of the KD. When the ketoacidosis did not improve, and the anion gap remained high despite hydration with IV fluids and subcutaneous insulin therapy, the endocrinology service was consulted. The endocrine team made the patient NPO and started an IV insulin drip with dextrose containing IV fluids per a standard DKA protocol. The anion gap normalized in <8 h.

The progression of the resolution of metabolic acidosis and plasma glucose during admission is summarized in Figure 18.1.

The patient improved and tolerated food intake after resolution of the acidosis. T1D was confirmed with positive GAD65 antibodies (<250 IU/mL). She was discharged home on basal-bolus insulin therapy with glargine and premeal aspart. She was also started on a continuous glucose monitor (CGM) to allow for early detection of hypoglycemia and scheduled for follow-up in our clinic. After 3 months, her HbA$_{1c}$ improved to 7.8% with no episodes of hypoglycemia.

Our patient presented with eDKA, which is a severe condition that presents with milder degrees of hyperglycemia than are typically seen in patients presenting with DKA (blood glucose <250 mg/dL). She had an anion gap metabolic acidosis with high ketone bodies.[1] The diagnosis of eDKA is challenging, since near-normal blood glucose levels can be misleading and precipitating factor(s) can be less apparent. The pathophysiology remains incompletely understood but has been described as occurring when there is insufficient carbohydrate intake causing starvation ketosis with activation of counterregulatory hormones in the context of an insulin-deficient state. Known precipitating factors for eDKA include prolonged fasting, pregnancy, pancreatitis, alcohol, cocaine intoxication, and sodium–glucose cotransporter 2 (SGLT2) inhibitors, among others. The development of eDKA while on a KD has not been well characterized in patients with diabetes.

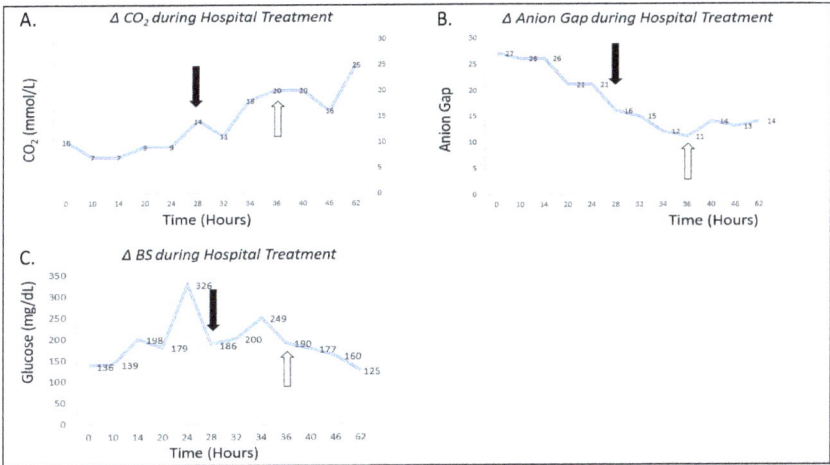

Figure 18.1—Graphic representation of serum changes during hospital treatment of eDKA. *A:* Change in CO_2 (mmol/L) in serum. *B:* Change in anion gap. *C:* Change in serum glucose. Black arrows represent initial NPO, insulin drip intervention. White arrows represent point of transition to basal and bolus insulin and initiation of carbohydrate-consistent diet (60 g per meal).

The American Diabetes Association (ADA) offers dietary recommendations as part of medical nutrition therapy, but the ideal diet remains controversial and varies among different patients.[2] Over the past years, the KD has gained popularity as a weight loss strategy. In patients with diabetes, a KD has been advocated as a way of decreasing postprandial hyperglycemia. Patients on these diets ingest low-carbohydrate, high-fat meals producing metabolic changes similar to what can occur with starvation. Metabolic needs are met by breaking down fat, resulting in the generation of ketone bodies, which contributes to metabolic acidosis.[3] KD leads to depletion of glycogen stores with a low insulin-to-glucagon ratio. These diets can also contribute to dehydration, hepatic steatosis, worsening insulin resistance, and impaired insulin secretion due in part to the low carbohydrate content.

In our patient, while the KD successfully contributed to her weight loss, it also put her in a nutritional ketotic state with more "normal" blood glucose levels and dehydration. The concurrent use of the SGLT2 inhibitor exacerbated the dehydration by decreasing glucose reabsorption in the proximal convoluted tubules of the nephron, causing glucosuria and promoting osmotic water loss. Concurrent use of the SGLT2 inhibitor amplified the ketone body production, thus precipitating ketoacidosis.[4]

There is an increased frequency in off-label use of SGLT2 inhibitors in patients with T1D. Some studies showed improvements in patient-reported outcomes or quality of life, with less hypoglycemia or greater time in range as assessed by CGM.[4] When added to insulin therapy, overall HbA_{1c} improvement is in the range of 0.3–0.5%, but with an apparent dose-dependent increase in risk of DKA ranging from 2% up to 5%.[5] Following early reports of eDKA with SGLT inhibitors,[1] the U.S. Food and Drug Administration as well as the European Medicine Agency did not approve the use of these agents for patients with T1D. Some experts suggest that this risk can be diminished by the use of basal insulin and proper hydration.[4,5] Even though our patient continued basal insulin, she still developed ketoacidosis. When she reached the point of higher ketone body–to–insulin ratio, she developed early symptoms of DKA with decreased appetite and nausea that over time led to dehydration and eventually full-blown eDKA.

Diabetes management requires the correct characterization of the patient's underlying disorder, followed by individualization of medical therapy. In her case, she was of normal weight with a T1D phenotype and without cardiovascular disease. Neither a KD nor SGLT2 inhibitors should have been prescribed for this patient. Until large-scale, randomized controlled trials are conducted to assess the safety and efficacy of KD in patients with T1D, recommending extreme low-carbohydrate dietary approaches for glycemic control and weight loss, especially to older patients who may be more susceptible to dehydration, should be discouraged. The take-home message here is that clinicians should avoid KDs in patients with T1D as well as the use of SGLT2 inhibitors, given the risk of tipping patients into eDKA, as occurred in our case.

COMMENTARY

This case brings attention to several important issues. One is that many older adult patients are inappropriately diagnosed and treated as if they have type 2 diabetes. Another issue is the description of several potential precipitating factors for eDKA, defined as DKA occurring with only mild elevations in blood glucose levels. This patient had several potential causes for eDKA, any one of which could have precipitated her presentation. One is the prescription for a KD that was used to treat type 1 diabetes before the discovery of insulin that is now more frequently used as a weight loss strategy without definitive evidence for efficacy. Another precipitating factor for the DKA in this patient was the addition of an SGLT2 inhibitor. These agents are known to be associated with an increase in risk for eDKA in patients with type 2 diabetes as well as type 1 diabetes, particularly during periods of fasting, such as preparation for surgery or other procedures. This patient case emphasizes the need for caution in patient selection and education when prescribing these agents.

Mary Korytkowski, MD

REFERENCES

1. Peters AL, Buschur EO, Buse JB, Cohan P, Diner JC, Hirsch IB. Euglycemic diabetic ketoacidosis: a potential complication of treatment with sodium–glucose cotransporter 2 inhibition. *Diabetes Care* 2015;38:1687–1693

2. American Diabetes Association. 5. Facilitating behavior change and well-being to improve health outcomes: *Standard of Medical Care in Diabetes—2020. Diabetes Care* 2020;43(Suppl. 1):S48–S65. https://doi.org/10.2337/dc20-S005

3. Bolla AM, Caretto A, Laurenzi A, Scavini M, Piemoti L. Low-carb and ketogenic diets in type 1 and type 2 diabetes. *Nutrients* 2019:11:962. https://doi: 10.3390/nu11050962

4. Danne T, Garg S, Peters AL, et al. International consensus on risk management of diabetes ketoacidosis in patients with type 1 diabetes treated with sodium–glucose cotransporter (SGLT) inhibitors. *Diabetes Care* 2019;42: 1147–1154. https:// doi:10.2337/dc18-2316

5. Lu J, Tang L, Meng H, Zhao J, Liang Y. Effects of sodium-glucose cotransporter (SGLT) inhibitors in addition to insulin therapy on glucose control and safety outcomes with type 1 diabetes: a meta-analysis of randomized controlled trials. *Diabetes Metab Res Rev* 2019;35:e3169. https://doi:10.1002/dmrr.3169

Part 3

Cancer Therapy and Diabetes

Case 19

Immune Checkpoint Inhibitor–Induced Type 1 Diabetes

Halis Kaan Akturk, MD,[1] and Aaron W. Michels, MD[1]

A 64-year-old Caucasian male with no previous history of diabetes presented with nausea, vomiting, fatigue, increased urination, and thirst over the 3 days before presentation, along with worsening of his mental status. He was being treated with pembrolizumab (monoclonal antibody targeting programmed cell death receptor-1 [PD-1]) infusions for advanced lung cancer. His most recent dose was 3 days before presentation, and his first dose was 24 days prior. He had a normal BMI (24.8 kg/m²), and the only pertinent past medical history was hypertension before the diagnosis of lung cancer. He has a 40–pack-year history of smoking. He had not been treated with glucocorticoids recently. His lab results at presentation showed significant hyperglycemia (glucose of 680 mg/dL) with anion gap metabolic acidosis, consistent with severe diabetic ketoacidosis (DKA) (arterial pH of 7.1, bicarbonate level of 4 mEq/L, β-hydroxybutyrate level of 28 mmol/L, anion gap of 26) and HbA$_{1c}$ of 6.9%. His HbA$_{1c}$ was 5.8% before the initiation of pembrolizumab therapy, and he had normal fasting glucose results before each infusion. On physical exam, he was found to be tachypneic and confused with significant distress. He was admitted to the intensive care unit and treated with intravenous (IV) fluids, electrolytes, and insulin. On further investigation, he had high titers of GAD65 antibodies, 218 (0–20 DK units), and a low C-peptide level of 0.2 (0.5–2 ng/mL). After 2 days in the intensive care unit, he was discharged on a regimen of multiple daily injections of insulin consisting of insulin glargine and lispro.

The emergence of cancer immunotherapy has revolutionized cancer treatment, but it can be associated with serious immune-related adverse effects, many of which affect endocrine organs. Immune checkpoints operate to halt an immune response to ensure that the immune system does not harm the host when reacting to a foreign protein (e.g., one of the mechanisms by which autoimmune diseases are avoided). Cancer cells have developed many mechanisms to evade the immune system with the cell surface expression of immune checkpoints as one of these. Monoclonal antibodies have been developed to inhibit immune checkpoints to enable an individual's immune cells to target cancer cells. Immune checkpoint inhibitors (ICIs) are state-of-the-art cancer immunotherapies used in many advanced cancers in adult and pediatric patients.

[1]Barbara Davis Center for Diabetes, University of Colorado, Aurora, Colorado.

DOI: 10.2337/9781580407663.19

ICI-induced type 1 diabetes has been reported with both inhibitors of anti–PD-1 and its ligand PD-L1. Pembrolizumab is a PD-1 inhibitor that is given every 3 weeks by IV infusion. In our case, pembrolizumab caused a sudden onset of diabetic ketoacidosis 4 weeks after the initial dose.

In large medical centers, the incidence of ICI-induced type 1 diabetes has been reported between 0.9 to 1.8%.[1,2] This incidence is much higher than that in spontaneous diabetes that develops in children and adults, which is ~0.3%. Most cases (~70%) of ICI-induced type 1 diabetes present in the first 90 days after the initial exposure to therapy.[2] About half of cases present with type 1 diabetes–associated antibodies (GAD65 antibodies) at presentation.[2] Patients presenting with type 1 diabetes–associated antibodies have a more rapid onset and higher incidence of diabetic ketoacidosis than those without antibodies.[2] HLA risk genes for type 1 diabetes, especially HLA-DR4, are associated with ICI-induced type 1 diabetes.[1,2] C-peptide levels are very low or absent at the presentation and reflect a rapid destruction of pancreatic β-cells. Notable in this case was the fact that the patient had a normal fasting blood glucose 3 days before presenting with DKA. Lack of a honeymoon phase and lower HbA_{1c} at presentation are classic findings of ICI-induced type 1 diabetes and may be explained by the increase in blood glucose in a short period of time. In some cases, rapid reduction in pancreas volume and increase in pancreatic enzymes (amylase and lipase) have also been reported, suggesting generalized pancreas inflammation.

Insulin-requiring diabetes is permanent, and the treatment of diabetes is not different than prototypical type 1 diabetes that develops in children and young adults.[3] Unlike the treatment of other immune-related adverse events after ICI therapy, steroids are not effective and worsen diabetes management. Considering the increasing indications and use of ICIs, health care providers and patients receiving these therapies should be aware of the potential for this serious adverse event. Guidelines and risk assessment strategies need to be developed to identify and monitor patients at greater risk. Patients with known type 1 diabetes-associated antibodies and high-risk HLA genes may be monitored more thoroughly with frequent self-monitoring of blood glucose levels or use of continuous glucose monitors to prevent life-threatening diabetic ketoacidosis.

COMMENTARY

This is an interesting case of ICI-induced diabetes in a 64-year-old man with high titers of GAD65 antibodies, 218 (0–20 DK units), and a low C-peptide level, 0.2 (0.5–2 ng/mL). Unfortunately, this case is not unique, and with greater use of this anti-cancer therapy, most oncologists and diabetologists have encountered such patients in their practice. This presentation properly concludes that treatment of patients with ICI-induced diabetes is not different from type 1 diabetes and requires insulin therapy.

Anne Peters, MD

REFERENCES

1. Stamatouli AM, Quandt Z, Perdigoto AL, et al. Collateral damage: insulin-dependent diabetes induced with checkpoint inhibitors. *Diabetes* 2018;67:1471–1480

2. Akturk HK, Kahramangil D, Sarwal A, et al. Immune checkpoint inhibitor-induced type 1 diabetes: a systematic review and meta-analysis. *Diabet Med* 2019;36:1075–1081

3. Akturk HK, Michels AW. Adverse events associated with immune checkpoint blockade. *N Engl J Med* 2018;378:1163–1164

Case 20

Partial β-Cell Destruction: An Atypical Case of Immune Checkpoint Inhibitor Diabetes

Zoe Quandt, MD,[1] Paras Mehta, MD,[1] Katy K. Tsai, MD,[2]
Victoria Hsiao, MD,[1] and Robert J. Rushakoff, MD[1]

A 50-year-old woman was started on adjuvant pembrolizumab for stage IIIC melanoma after surgery. She had no prior history of diabetes, thyroid disease, or other autoimmune disease. Pre-infusion random blood glucose levels were 84–105 mg/dL. After 36 weeks, she developed hypothyroidism (thyroid-stimulating hormone [TSH] 17.5 [0.5–4.1 μIU/L], free T-4 6 [10–18 μg/dL]), and started levothyroxine. Pembrolizumab was continued. For 9 weeks after her diagnosis with immune checkpoint inhibitor (ICI)-induced hypothyroidism, her pre-infusion random blood glucose levels ranged from 102 to 133 mg/dL. At 45 weeks (15 cycles) after initiating pembrolizumab, her random blood glucose level was 260 mg/dL. She was not on glucocorticoids and had no other signs of inflammation or stress. Pembrolizumab was continued. Just before her 17th cycle, 48 weeks after initiating adjuvant pembrolizumab, her random blood glucose level was 482 mg/dL with a normal anion gap and bicarbonate level, and her HbA_{1c} was 8.9%. Her last dose of pembrolizumab was held. She started metformin and liraglutide. In just 3 weeks, a random C-peptide was inadequate at 1.7 ng/mL (0.8–3.5 ng/mL) with a recent random blood glucose level of 220 mg/dL and HbA_{1c} of 10.3%, showing the acuity and extremity of her hyperglycemia. Over the course of the following year, she achieved excellent glucose control (HbA_{1c} 6.3–7.1%) on this regimen with preservation of insulin production (C-peptide levels of 1.4–1.8, with matched random blood glucose of 92–129 mg/dL). She never required insulin. Her family history includes a sister with hyperthyroidism of unknown etiology and a father with adult-onset, diet-controlled diabetes. Her physical exam at diabetes diagnosis was notable for a BMI of 33.3 kg/m² and no acanthosis nigricans. Her β-cell autoantibodies and thyroid autoantibodies were negative, and her HLA type was DR3-DQ2/DR3-DQ-2.

Autoimmune diabetes caused by immune checkpoint inhibitors (ICIs) is rare, occurring in ~1% of patients exposed to this form of cancer immunotherapy. Typically, this immune-related adverse event occurs after treatment

[1]Division of Endocrinology and Metabolism. [2]Division of Hematology/Oncology, University of California, San Francisco, California.

DOI: 10.2337/9781580407663.20

with PD-1/PD-L1 inhibitors. It is characterized by abrupt insulinopenia leading to acute hyperglycemia. β-Cell autoantibodies are positive in approximately
half the cases. DKA is common at the time of diagnosis. Recovery of β-cell
function has been reported in only two case reports.[1] In one case, spontaneous
resolution occurred after cessation of ICI therapy in a patient who had not
fully lost insulin production[2] and, in the other, the patient, who again had not
fully lost insulin production, was treated with infliximab for concurrent inflammatory arthritis before resolution of ICI-induced diabetes.[3] This is a case of
ICI-induced diabetes (Figure 20.1) in which the patient did not have complete
loss of β-cell function. The acuity of her hyperglycemia is not consistent with
new-onset type 2 diabetes. At diagnosis, her C-peptide was inadequate, suggesting insufficient insulin production rather than insulin resistance. Therefore, her hyperglycemia is more consistent with ICI-induced diabetes than
type 2 diabetes. Furthermore, her HLA type confers high risk for developing
T1D. Her autoantibodies were not positive, which is common in ICI-induced
diabetes. Atypically, she did not progress to fulminant β-cell failure, which
could have been due to cessation of pembrolizumab (although ICI cessation is
not unique to this case), initiation of liraglutide (a glucagon-like peptide-1
[GLP-1] agonist) and metformin, or other unknown immunologic responses
that inhibited full β-cell loss. While liraglutide was not necessarily chosen for
this reason, GLP-1 agonists have been proposed to help preserve β-cell health
and have been seen to restore euglycemia in combination with gastrin in

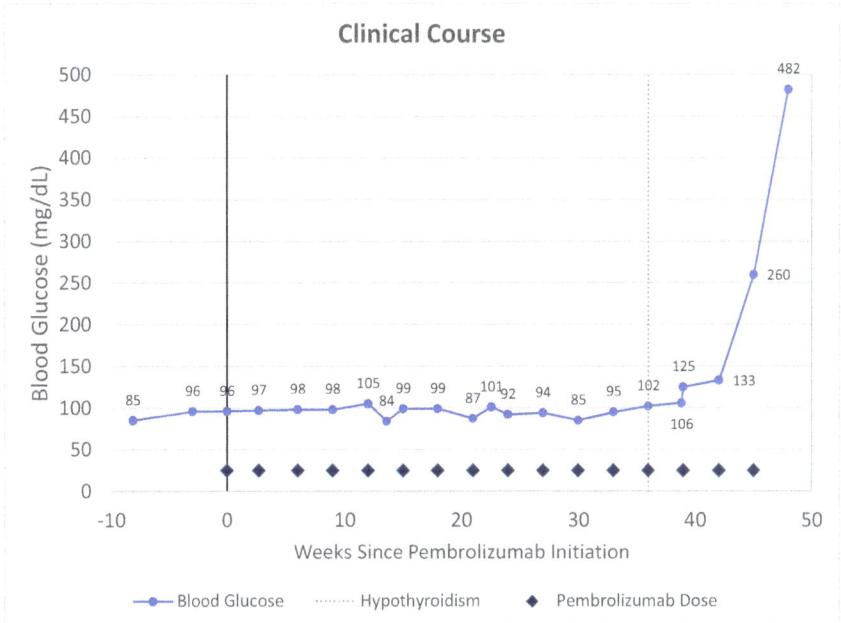

Figure 20.1—Effect of pembrolizumab on blood glucose levels.

diabetic-prone mice. While liraglutide is still a daily injection, it is far easier to manage than the basal-bolus regimens required for type 1 diabetes and more typical ICI-induced diabetes. This case raises the possibility of preventing fully insulin-dependent ICI-induced diabetes if hyperglycemia is caught early, emphasizing the importance of ongoing vigilant safety monitoring through CPI course and timely consultation with endocrinology.

COMMENTARY

This is another excellent case illustrating the ability of ICIs to destroy pancreatic β-cells and cause diabetes. Unlike the previous case, however, pembrolizumab did not cause a complete destruction of β-cell function, and the patient maintained reasonable glycemia on metformin and liraglutide. This result may be partially explained because pembrolizumab was discontinued. Another interesting and not so uncommon point of this case is that this patient also developed hypothyroidism. Overall, close glucose monitoring in cancer patients treated with ICIs should be standard in practice.

Anne Peters, MD

REFERENCES

1. Quandt Z, Young A, Anderson M. 2020. Immune checkpoint inhibitor diabetes mellitus: a novel form of autoimmune diabetes. *Clin Exp Immunol* 2020;200:1–10

2. Hansen E, Sahasrabudhe D, Sievert L. A case report of insulin-dependent diabetes as immune-related toxicity of pembrolizumab: presentation, management and outcome. *Cancer Immunol Immunother* 2016;65:765–767

3. Trinh B, Donath MY, Läubli H. Successful treatment of immune checkpoint inhibitor–induced diabetes with infliximab. *Diabetes Care* 2019;42:e153–e154

Case 21

Checkpoint Inhibitor–Induced Diabetes

Paras Mehta, MD,[1] Zoe Quandt, MD,[1] and Robert J. Rushakoff, MD[1]

A 70-year-old Asian woman with unresectable lung adenocarcinoma was referred for abnormal thyroid function tests and hyperglycemia. She had no personal or family history of thyroid disease, hyperglycemia, or autoimmune disorders. Five months before referral, she began durvalumab, a U.S. Food and Drug Administration (FDA)-approved immunotherapy targeting the ligand for programmed cell death receptor (PD)-1 for her lung cancer. One week before referral, she was noted to have a thyroid-stimulating hormone of 20.55 vIU/L (reference 0.4–4.5) and free T4 of 11 pmol/L (reference 10–18) and was started on levothyroxine for presumed hypothyroidism related to immunotherapy. At that time, her random glucose was 217 mg/dL. She subsequently developed polyuria and polydipsia, and when seen in the endocrine clinic, her HbA$_{1c}$ was 7.3%. C-peptide was 1.0 ng/mL (0.8–3.5) with concurrent glucose of 317 mg/dL, and islet autoantibodies (GAD65, islet cell antibody [ICA]-512, insulin, and zinc transporter 8) were all negative. She was diagnosed with immune checkpoint inhibitor (ICI)-induced diabetes, received diabetes education, and was started initially on lispro with a carbohydrate ratio of 1 to 15. This initial clinic visit took several hours. One week later, she returned to clinic and was started on basal insulin with 4 units glargine at night. Her immunotherapy was held and adenocarcinoma remained stable on imaging. Since her diagnosis of ICI-induced diabetes, she has been evaluated in the endocrine clinic at least 1 to 2 times per month. Six months after ICI-induced diabetes diagnosis, her HbA$_{1c}$ was 8.4%, glargine was increased to 7 units, and continuous glucose monitoring had been initiated.

ICI-induced diabetes is a rare endocrine side effect and occurs in ~1% of patients on ICIs.[1-4] It is seen almost exclusively in PD-1 or its ligand, PD-L1, inhibitor therapy and likely occurs because of disinhibition of T-cells. The diagnosis is considered to be likely if a patient on immunotherapy (without a prior known diagnosis of diabetes or impaired glucose tolerance) develops severe hyperglycemia with a low corresponding C-peptide level or presents in diabetic ketoacidosis (DKA).

[1]Division of Endocrinology and Metabolism, University of California, San Francisco, California.

DOI: 10.2337/9781580407663.21

Several clinical characteristics can help differentiate ICI-induced diabetes from autoimmune type 1 diabetes or latent autoimmune diabetes in adults (LADA). Patients are generally older (median age 60–70 years in several studies), likely reflecting the population with advanced cancer. The development of hyperglycemia and β-cell dysfunction is relatively acute, which is evident by the discordance between plasma glucose values (often 300–1,000 mg/dL) and HbA$_{1c}$ (usually around 8%, indicating a 3-month glucose average between 180 and 190 mg/dL) at diagnosis. Additionally, only approximately half of patients are found to have islet autoantibodies at the time of diagnosis. While initially hypothesized that autoantibodies would develop over the course of the disease, longer-term data have shown that those who are initially negative rarely develop autoantibodies. The features of ICI-induced diabetes are actually most similar to the fulminant form of type 1 diabetes described in Asian populations in the 2000s, in which rapid β-cell destruction occurs in a matter of weeks with negative islet autoantibodies.

Given that many patients present with DKA and nearly all are insulinopenic, the mainstay of ICI-induced diabetes treatment is insulin. This finding presents a significant practical challenge and burden to a patient population already dealing with an advanced malignancy, frequent visits to an oncologist and infusion center, and glucocorticoid treatment at times. Immediate insulin initiation and diabetes education are needed, along with close clinical follow-up. The extent of diabetes education and follow-up interval should be determined on a case-by-case basis. In our patient described above, insulin initiation was accomplished in a stepwise fashion, with bolus and basal insulin being introduced 1 week apart. In the future, we hope to develop diabetes education programs specific to ICI-induced diabetes, given the increasing use of immunotherapy and corresponding increase in cases of ICI-induced diabetes.

One additional challenge is the decision regarding continuation of immunotherapy. No definitive guidelines exist, and this should be evaluated on a case-by-case basis as well. Although better understanding of the underlying pathophysiology is needed, we believe that the β-cell destruction in ICI-induced diabetes is likely irreversible (and may be reversible if caught exceedingly early on, when C-peptide levels are still detectable, but that result has not been shown to date). There is likely to be minimal benefit in holding immunotherapy solely for ICI-induced diabetes. Other factors should be considered, such as additional immune-related adverse events and the oncologic response to immunotherapy. In our patient, given that she had two adverse events (hypothyroidism and hyperglycemia) with minimal residual disease, the decision was made to pause immunotherapy. Fortunately, the decision to continue to hold immunotherapy has remained straightforward, since her cancer has not progressed.

In summary, ICI-induced diabetes is a distinct form of diabetes that manifests with rapid β-cell destruction, long-term insulin dependence, and variable detectable autoimmunity in the setting of PD-1 or PD-L1 inhibitor treatment. Effective management requires close clinical follow-up and focused diabetes education to assist an already-burdened patient population.

COMMENTARY

Immunotherapy for cancer has entered the mainstream of therapeutic interventions in clinical oncology. Diabetes is an unfortunate side effect of this promising therapy. Both PD-1 and PD-L1 inhibitors are known for this side effect. Hypothyroidism is another common side effect of ICIs. Interestingly, in this case, treating physicians elected to start therapy with mealtime insulin, adding basal insulin 1 week later. Most commonly, this sequence is reversed and basal insulin is started before mealtime insulin. These details notwithstanding, insulin therapy appears to be the proper treatment of this condition, which in all respects is identical to type 1 diabetes.

Anne Peters, MD

REFERENCES

1. Quandt Z, Young A, Anderson M. Immune checkpoint inhibitor diabetes mellitus: a novel form of autoimmune diabetes. *Clin Exp Immunol* 2020;200:131–140

2. Kotwal A, Haddox C, Block M, Kudva YC. Immune checkpoint inhibitors: an emerging cause of insulin-dependent diabetes. *BMJ Open Diabetes Res Care* 2019;7:e000591

3. Wright JJ, Salem J, Johnson DB, et al. Increased reporting of immune checkpoint inhibitor–associated diabetes. *Diabetes Care* 2018;41:e150–e151

4. Hanafusa T, Imagawa A. Fulminant type 1 diabetes: a novel clinical entity requiring special attention by all medical practitioners. *Nat Clin Pract Endocrinol Metab* 2007;3:36–45

Case 22

Alpelisib-Induced Hyperglycemia: A Case Series

Richa Patel, MD,[1] Ana Ramirez Berlioz, MD,[1] Amber Pinson, MD, [1] and Michael Gardner, MD[1]

C ase 1, a 62-year-old female with recurrent invasive ductal carcinoma metastatic to lung and bone, was referred to Endocrinology for management of hyperglycemia. She was initially diagnosed with breast cancer in 1996 and underwent bilateral mastectomy. She remained cancer-free until 2018, when biopsy of a new right chest wall lump confirmed invasive ductal carcinoma. Gene testing of the tumor revealed PIK3CA mutation and once-daily alpelisib therapy was begun. Pre-chemotherapy HbA_{1c} was 5.6%, but within a few weeks of starting therapy, fasting hyperglycemia of up to 160 mg/dL was noted. Given persistent hyperglycemia and symptoms of dry mouth and polydipsia, twice-daily metformin therapy was started. Pronounced evening hyperglycemia persisted, and the dose of metformin was increased.

Case 2, a 47-year-old female with history of major depressive disorder, generalized anxiety disorder, and recurrent metastatic breast cancer, was referred to Endocrinology for management of alpelisib-induced diabetes. Breast cancer had progressed despite conventional chemotherapy and hormonal therapy. Alpelisib therapy was started after genetic testing confirmed PIK3CA mutation. Within 12 weeks of starting alpelisib, HbA_{1c} increased from 5.1 to 6.9%. She had persistent hyperglycemia and reported fasting blood glucose of 442 mg/dL. Metformin-sitagliptin combination therapy was started, with significant improvement in hyperglycemia. Unfortunately, alpelisib was eventually stopped because of disease progression, and the patient was subsequently lost to follow-up.

Case 3, a 59-year-old female with metastatic invasive ductal carcinoma, gastroesophageal reflux disease, and chronic low back pain, was diagnosed with alpelisib-induced diabetes. Despite excellent structural response to the drug, the dose had to be reduced because of significant hyperglycemia and rash. Upon initial evaluation by Endocrinology, the patient was noted to have fasting hyperglycemia ranging from 120–200 mg/dL, with HbA_{1c} of 5.1%. Metformin was started because of worsening hyperglycemia despite lifestyle modifications. About 12 weeks later, she was admitted with significant hyperglycemia of 432 mg/dL and an HbA_{1c} of 9.1%. No

[1]Department of Medicine, Division of Endocrinology and Metabolism, University of Missouri–Columbia, Columbia, Missouri.

 DOI: 10.2337/9781580407663.22

hyperosmolality or ketosis was noted. She was treated with intravenous (IV) insulin therapy during hospital admission and was discharged home on a regimen of metformin and basal insulin. She remained on this regimen for a few weeks, but because of persistent nausea, metformin therapy was discontinued. Because of concerns that insulin would decrease the effectiveness of alpelisib, canagliflozin was added and insulin was titrated off. The patient was also started on a low-carbohydrate diet, resulting in well-controlled blood glucose. She continues to have excellent response to alpelisib therapy.

Hyperglycemia associated with alpelisib therapy is an on-target effect due to phosphatidylinositol 3-kinase (PI3K) inhibition. The PI3K signaling pathway has key effects on an array of cellular functions including growth, differentiation, cytoskeletal rearrangement, and cell survival and plays an important role in insulin action. Class I PI3K consists of a catalytic subunit p110 (p110α, p110β, p110γ, p110δ) and a regulatory subunit p85.[1] P110α isoform (encoded by the PIK3CA gene) is frequently mutated in cancers. Inhibitors of PI3K have therefore emerged as promising therapy in treating cancers. Alpelisib (Piqray) is one such drug that inhibits the PI3K p110α isoform. It was approved by the FDA in 2019 for treatment of hormone receptor–positive, human epidermal growth factor receptor 2 (HER2)-negative, advanced or metastatic breast cancer with the PIK3CA mutation. Hyperglycemia, resulting from hampered metabolic actions of insulin at different levels, is one of the most common side effects of this drug, since PI3K plays a central role in insulin signaling in multiple tissues including liver (preventing glycogenolysis), skeletal muscles (inhibiting glucose uptake), and adipocytes. Many cancers have an unusual dependence on glucose metabolism because of aerobic glycolysis (the Warburg effect) and the use of glucose and glutamine for building blocks.[2] Activating mutations in PI3K serve to supply this glucose and thus are a promising target for cancer therapy.

Insulin via its metabolic pathway activates PI3K and further activates AKT, which mobilizes GLUT4 to the cell surface allowing cellular glucose uptake. Thus, inhibition of PI3Ks leads to insulin resistance, glucose intolerance, and hyperinsulinemia. However, the specific roles of the different p110 isoforms remain elusive.

With advancements in cancer therapy, it is important to identify and address these metabolic derangements to minimize interruption of treatment. Hopkins et al.[3] showed in animal models that hyperglycemia after PI3K inhibitor therapy is transient, with compensatory hyperinsulinemia within a few hours of PI3K inhibition. This occurrence is thought to reactivate the PI3K/AKT signaling axis. In the above-mentioned study, response to sodium–glucose transporter 2 (SGLT2) inhibitor therapy and ketogenic diet was found to be superior when compared to metformin, also resulting in lower insulin levels.

In a phase 3 trial of alpelisib plus fulvestrant, hyperglycemia was the most frequent adverse event occurring at a rate of 36.6% in the treatment group; treatment was discontinued in 6.3% of patients because of severe hyperglycemia.[4] During this study, participants experiencing hyperglycemia were recommended lifestyle modifications in line with recommendations by the American

Diabetes Association. Metformin therapy was started for mild hyperglycemia, but more severe hyperglycemia resulted in treatment interruption requiring IV fluids and insulin.

Metformin remains the first choice of treatment in alpelisib-induced hyperglycemia because of its availability and safe side-effect profile. Based on the mechanism of action of alpelisib, data in animal models suggest that agents acting through the insulin-signaling pathways have a limited role in therapy. SGLT2 inhibitors, on the other hand, appear to be a promising therapeutic option, since they inhibit renal glucose reabsorption, thus working independently of the insulin pathway. However, clinicians should assess risk of ketoacidosis in patients using SGLT2 inhibitors, especially given the high risk of dehydration and possibility of frequent steroid use in this population.

COMMENTARY

These three interesting cases illustrate development of alpelisib-induced hyperglycemia in patients with metastatic breast cancer whose HbA_{1c} was normal before the therapy. Two patients developed striking hyperglycemia, with blood glucose levels exceeding 400 mg/dL.

Hyperglycemia is an expected on-target side effect of the PIK3 inhibitor alpelisib, an important addition to the breast cancer therapeutic armamentarium in a new era of personalized medicine. Patients with an activating mutation in the PI3K/AKT pathway are good candidates for this promising therapy. PI3K has both mitogenic (thus, tumorigenic) and metabolic action. The latter involves activation of GLUT4-dependent glucose transport in insulin-sensitive tissues. Even though it may or may not be involved in promoting glucose uptake in cancerous tissue (that may not be GLUT4-dependent), inhibition of this pathway in insulin-sensitive tissues blocks glucose uptake, resulting in hyperglycemia or further deterioration of existing diabetes.

While metformin and SGLT2 inhibitors are good options for therapy, in some cases, insulin should be used. Adequate doses of insulin should overcome the inhibitory effect of alpelisib in insulin target tissues, while it is not clear whether insulin effect on PI3K in the tumor interferes with the therapeutic action of alpelisib in a particular tumor.

The bottom line is that new medications directed at various steps in cellular signaling might and do interfere with hormonal actions that might use the same signaling molecules.

Boris Draznin, MD, PhD

REFERENCES

1. Zhao L, Vogt PK. Class I PI3K in oncogenic cellular transformation. *Oncogene* 2008;27:5486–5496. doi:10.1038/onc.2008.244

2. Vander Heiden M, Cantley L, Thompson C. Understanding the Warburg effect: the metabolic requirements of cell proliferation. *Science* 2009;324: 1029–1033

3. Hopkins BD, Pauli C, Du X, et al. Suppression of insulin feedback enhances the efficacy of PI3K inhibitors. *Nature* 2018;560:499–503. doi:10.1038/ s41586-018-0343-4

4. André F, Ciruelos E, Rubovszky G, et al. Alpelisib for PIK3CA-mutated, hormone receptor–positive advanced breast cancer. *N Engl J Med* 2019;380: 1929–1940

Phosphatidylinositol 3-Kinase (PI3K) Inhibitor–Induced Hyperglycemia

Sanjita B. Chittimoju, MD,[1] Sara M. Alexanian, MD,[1] and Katherine L. Modzelewski, MD[1]

A 61-year-old female with past medical history of prediabetes and infiltrating ductal carcinoma of the right breast with bone and lung metastases, status post-partial mastectomy and hormonal therapy, was referred for management of hyperglycemia. Her primary tumor was positive for the PIK3CA H1047R, P471L mutation, and she started palliative treatment with the novel phosphatidylinositol 3-kinase (PIK3) inhibitor alpelisib 300 mg daily and fulvestrant. One month later, she was started on metformin 500 mg daily for high random blood glucose (BG) levels. After 2 months on alpelisib, she was hospitalized for severe hyperglycemia with BG of 1,007 mg/dL and acute kidney injury but without hyperglycemic crisis. Alpelisib and metformin were discontinued, and she was treated with fluids and intravenous insulin. She was discharged on Humulin 50-50 mixed insulin 15 units twice daily after normalization of creatinine.

Three weeks later, she was noted to have postprandial hypoglycemia while off of alpelisib. The mixed insulin was changed to insulin glargine 10 units daily and metformin was resumed. Her fasting BG improved from around 140 mg/dL to around 100 mg/dL, and insulin was discontinued. Alpelisib was then reinitiated per guidelines at a lower dose of 250 mg daily.[1] Within 1 week, she had recurrence of fasting hyperglycemia and was restarted on insulin glargine 10 units daily. Her BG remained elevated and sitagliptin 100 mg daily was added, resulting in fasting BG ranging from 156 to 199 mg/dL. Her insulin glargine dose was then increased to 20 units daily with improvement in her fasting BG to 140–179 mg/dL. Glycemic patterns on the two doses of insulin glargine are shown in Figures 23.1 and 23.2. After glycemic control improved, her most recent restaging imaging showed improvement in her lung and bone metastases, indicating the continued efficacy of alpelisib.

After the discovery of PI3K in 1985, the PI3K/AKT signaling pathway was found to play a central role in cellular physiology, including in apoptosis, cell survival, cell cycle progression, and metabolism.[2] About 40% of patients with

---

[1]Section of Endocrinology, Diabetes and Nutrition, Boston Medical Center and Boston University School of Medicine, Boston, Massachusetts.

 DOI: 10.2337/9781580407663.23

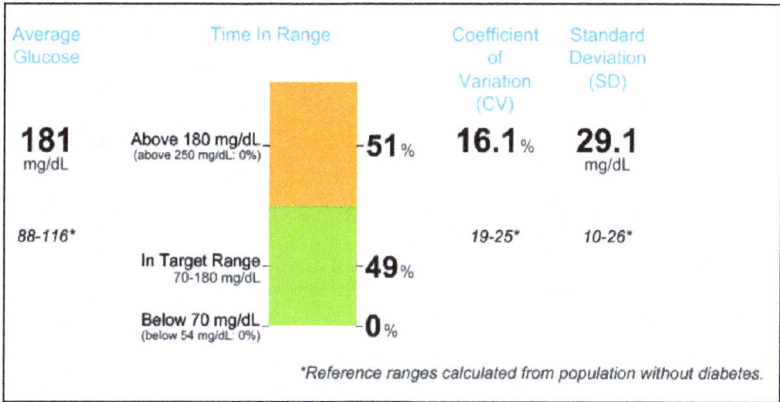

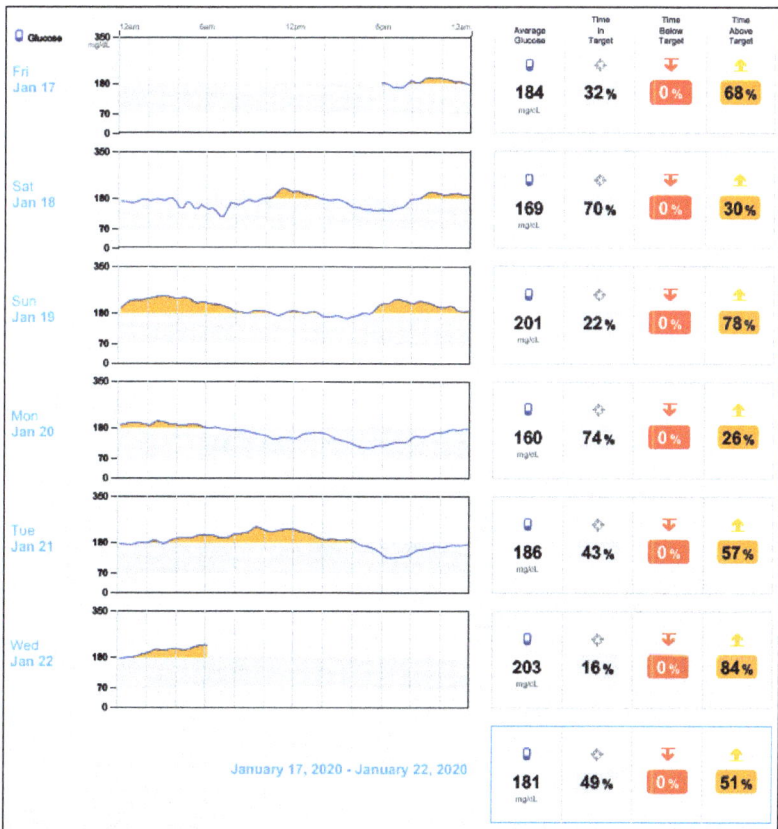

Figure 23.1—Glycemic control on insulin glargine 10 units daily using FreeStyle Libre–blinded continuous glucose monitoring (CGM).

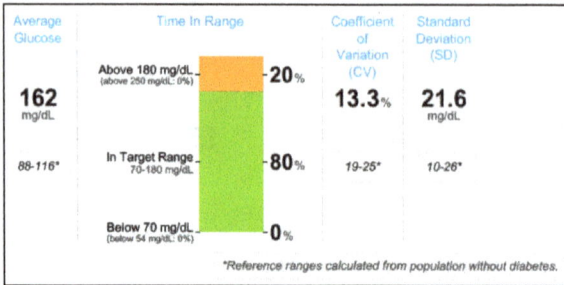

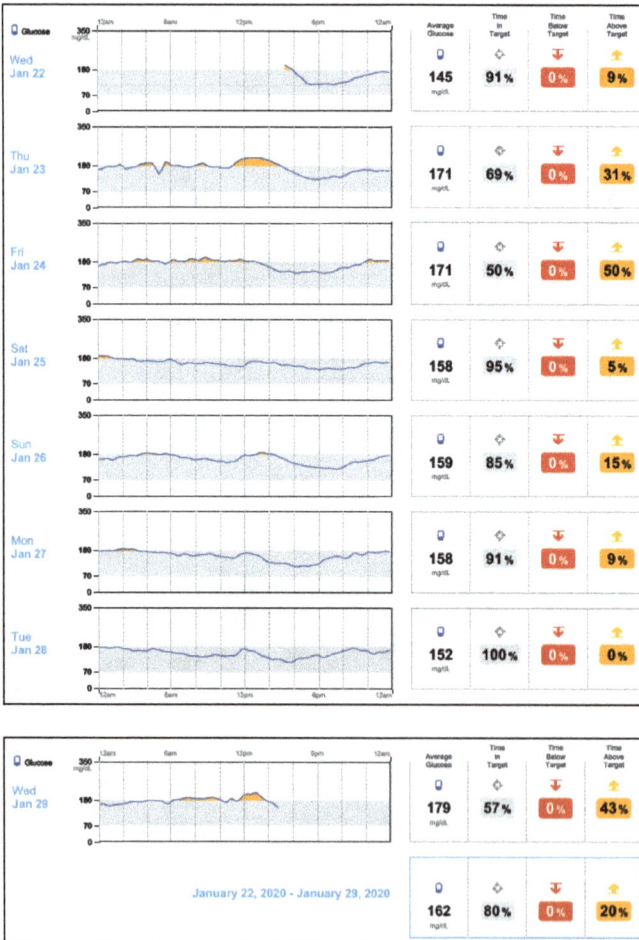

Figure 23.2—Glycemic control on insulin glargine 20 units daily using FreeStyle Libre–blinded CGM.

hormone receptor–positive, human epidermal growth factor receptor 2–negative breast cancer have activating mutations in the gene PIK3CA, which induces hyperactivation of an isoform of PI3K. Alpelisib, a PIK3 inhibitor, was recently approved in combination with fulvestrant as the first medication in this class for treating advanced breast cancer.

In the phase 3 randomized controlled trial (SOLAR-1) comparing alpelisib 300 mg daily with fulvestrant to placebo with fulvestrant, the alpelisib combination showed significantly improved progression-free survival in patients with PIK3CA mutation–positive breast cancer. However, the safety analysis demonstrated that 64% of the alpelisib group developed hyperglycemia, of which 32% had grade 3 hyperglycemia (>250–500 mg/dL) and 4% had grade 4 hyperglycemia (>500 mg/dL).[3]

In addition to its role in the cell cycle, the PI3K/AKT pathway is important for glucose homeostasis. Disruption leads to reduced glucose uptake, reduced glycogen synthesis, and increased glycolysis. These effects are generally seen within the first two cycles of treatment with alpelisib and are considered an "on target" effect. Although the hyperglycemia is thought to be transient in response to the activity of alpelisib, in individuals with impaired glucose metabolism, the effect can be significant and prolonged.[4] When choosing antihyperglycemic medications, consider medication safety, efficacy, and the potential in relation to the underlying malignancy. Insulin, a potent stimulator of PI3K signaling, could potentially have an undesired effect on tumor progression. In vitro animal studies have shown a compensatory increase in insulin release in mice in response to the hyperglycemia from PI3K inhibition, which may partially rescue PI3K signaling and could result in tumor progression.[5] The clinical relevance of this finding has not yet been defined in humans but raises concerns about exogenous insulin decreasing the efficacy of alpelisib. It has also been suggested that because PI3K inhibitors interfere with insulin action, exogenous insulin may not be effective, and use of insulin sensitizers may be preferable.

In the SOLAR-1 trial, metformin was used as first-line treatment for hyperglycemia, followed by pioglitazone and dipeptidyl peptidase-4 inhibitors.[3] Transient use of insulin was recommended if fasting blood glucose reached >250 mg/dL. For more symptomatic or higher-grade hyperglycemia, alpelisib could be held or the dose reduced. Our patient was not a good candidate for pioglitazone because of bone metastases that increased her risk for fracture and pedal edema. Sitagliptin was instead selected for its potential effect on postprandial hyperglycemia.

Some authors have advocated using sodium–glucose cotransporter 2 (SGLT2) inhibitors or ketogenic diets to manage hyperglycemia and reduce insulin levels in patients using PI3K inhibitors to decrease potential effects of insulin on tumor growth.[4] To date, these methods have not been studied in humans. Given the potential increased risk of diabetic ketoacidosis in ill, malnourished cancer patients, it is prudent to study these options in a controlled trial before recommending them in broad practice.

Because it has been postulated that exogenous insulin may be ineffective in patients using alpelisib because of its direct interference with cellular response to insulin, continuous glucose monitoring was used to monitor the effect of variable insulin doses. Glycemic control improved with a higher dose of insulin, suggesting that insulin is still efficacious in patients taking PI3K inhibitors. However, our understanding of the potential decrease in efficacy of alpelisib for cancer treatment in response to exogenous insulin is limited and potential reactivation of the PI3K-AKT pathway could be counter-productive.[5] In our patient, subsequent imaging showed improvement in her metastases, demonstrating continued efficacy of alpelisib, although so far only in short-term follow-up.

This case highlights that the mechanisms of hyperglycemia due to PI3K inhibition and its management are not well understood. More research is warranted to better understand how PI3K inhibitors affect glycemic control to help guide management. Additionally, while more research is needed on the potential reactivation of the PI3K-AKT pathway by exogenous insulin, insulin is effective in improving hyperglycemia and should be considered while closely monitoring for malignancy progression.

COMMENTARY

Personalized medicine is marching strong and oncology is the best example of its success. With identification of various mutations, the scientists have developed drugs attacking these specific mutations causing tumors in the first place. Activating mutations in the PI3 kinase/AKT pathway have been found in approximately one-third of all human cancers. This pathway is critical for the cell cycle: apoptosis, DNA repair, cellular senescence, angiogenesis, and cellular metabolism. Activating mutations in this pathway are associated with carcinogenesis and tumor angiogenesis. This is why a search for inhibitors of this pathway has been so active and fruitful in many situations.

Unfortunately, inhibition of PI3K/AKT pathway can also elicit substantial side effects, a long list of which is headed by hyperglycemia. The reason for this is that, in the insulin-sensitive tissues, such as skeletal muscle and adipose, GLUT4-dependent glucose uptake is under control of the PI3-K/AKT pathway. Thus, inhibition of this pathway will lead to impaired glucose uptake with resultant hyperglycemia. In a patient who already manifests glucose intolerance, this can be especially problematic.

This particular case illustrates both the appearance of severe hyperglycemia in a patient taking a novel PI3K pathway inhibitor and approach to mitigation of this side effect. Most likely, because inhibition of this pathway by alpelisib is not complete, higher doses of insulin can still activate PI3K/AKT in sensitive tissues to facilitate glucose uptake. Insulin sensitizers might work, but in my view, one might need higher doses of insulin to overcome inhibition of this pathway.

Boris Draznin, MD, PhD

REFERENCES

1. Goldman JW, Mendenhall MA, Rettinger SR. Hyperglycemia associated with targeted oncologic treatment: mechanisms and management. *Oncologist* 2016;21:1326–1336

2. Huang X, Liu G, Su Z. The PI3K/AKT pathway in obesity and type 2 diabetes. *Int J Biol Sci* 2018;14:1483–1496

3. André F, Ciruelos E, Rubovszky G, et al. Alpelisib for *PIK3CA*-mutated, hormone receptor–positive advanced breast cancer. *N Engl J Med* 2019;380; 1929–1940

4. Goncalves MD, Hopkins BD, Cantley LC. Phosphatidylinositol 3-kinase, growth disorders, and cancer. *N Engl J Med* 2018;379:2052–2062

5. Hopkins BD, Pauli C, Du X, et al. Suppression of insulin feedback enhances the efficacy of PI3K inhibitors. *Nature* 2018;560:499–503

Part 4

Autoimmunity and Diabetes

Misleading Diabetes: A Case of Type B Insulin Resistance Associated With Lupus Nephritis and Autoimmune Hepatitis

Ghada Elshimy,[1*] Mary Esquivel,[2*] Meredith McFarland,[2] Jessica Ricciuto,[2] Christopher Tessier,[2] Joanna Miragaya,[2] and Ricardo Correa, MD, EdD, FACP, FACE, FAPCR, CMQ [1,2]

ACKNOWLEDGMENTS

The authors thank Benjamin Gigliotti and Jose Flores from the Division of Endocrinology, Massachusetts General Hospital, Harvard Medical School, Boston MA; Robert Semple, Laboratory at the University of Cambridge; and Rebecca Brown and Elaine Cochran, National Institute of Diabetes and Digestive and Kidney Diseases, National Institutes of Health, Bethesda, MD.

A 20-year-old African American woman with a history of presumed type 2 diabetes on 16 units of insulin daily (0.27 units/kg) and metformin (her last HbA_{1c} was 13% despite compliance to medications), mixed connective tissue disease, and hypothyroidism presented with seizure-like activity. She had no family history of endocrine or autoimmune diseases. On initial laboratory workup, she was hyperglycemic with blood glucose (BG) of 627 mg/dL. The remaining workup is described in Tables 24.1 and 24.2. Because of progressive hyperglycemia refractory to subcutaneous insulin, insulin drip was initiated and titrated up to 60 units/h (total daily dose of 1,560 units). The specific workup showed a C-peptide level of 11.16 ng/mL with total insulin level >1,500 IU/L while transiently off the insulin infusion. Other causes of hyperglycemia, including 24-h urine-free cortisol, impaired fasting glucose (IGF)-1, and insulin antibody, were all negative or within normal limits. Additionally, she had acute kidney injury due to lupus nephritis confirmed by kidney biopsy and had autoimmune hepatitis confirmed by liver biopsy. Interestingly, blood glucose significantly improved after the first dose of pulse steroid therapy ordered by nephrology, with decreased insulin requirement to 10 units/h. However, this effect was transient and insulin requirements increased back up

[1]Division of Endocrinology, University of Arizona College of Medicine, Phoenix, Arizona. [2]Division of Endocrinology, Warren Alpert Medical School of Brown University, Providence, Rhode Island.
*G.E. and M.E. contributed equally as first coauthors.

DOI: 10.2337/9781580407663.24 **97**

Table 24.1—Laboratory testing on admission

Laboratory test	Results
Blood glucose	627 mg/dL
Sodium	122 mEq/L
Bicarbonate	20 mEq/L
Anion gap	6
Creatinine	2.3 mg/dL
Glomerular filtration rate	27 mL/min/1.73 m²
β-Hydroxybutyrate	0.3 mmol/L
Urine analysis	Negative for ketones
Venous blood gas pH	7.36

to 60 units/h once the steroids were weaned. Over the next few days, she was then transitioned to a high dose of U-500 pending remaining laboratory workup results. Because of suspicion for an insulin receptor disorder, further workup was performed. Adiponectin level was elevated at 42 λg/mL (0.8–3.85 ng/mL). While awaiting results of insulin receptor antibody testing, the patient was started on a sodium–glucose cotransporter 2 (SGLT2) inhibitor in addition to the U-500. The requirements for insulin decreased as presented in Figures 24.1 and 24.2. Insulin receptor antibody titers (AIRAs) later returned positive (Figure 24.3). The diagnosis of type B insulin resistance (TBIR) was confirmed. Subsequently, a National Institutes of Health protocol with rituximab, cyclophosphamide, and pulse-dose steroids was started, and remission was achieved after two cycles (3 months later) (Figures 24.1 and 24.2).

TBIR is a rare autoimmune disorder that causes glucose level abnormalities due to polyclonal autoantibodies (usually immunoglobulin G) produced

Table 24.2—Laboratory testing the day before admission

Laboratory test	Results
Alanine aminotransferase	679 IU/L
Aspartate aminotransferase	856 IU/L
Alkaline phosphatase	459 IU/L
Total testosterone	130 ng/dL
HbA$_{1c}$	13.9% (9.5% 6 months prior)

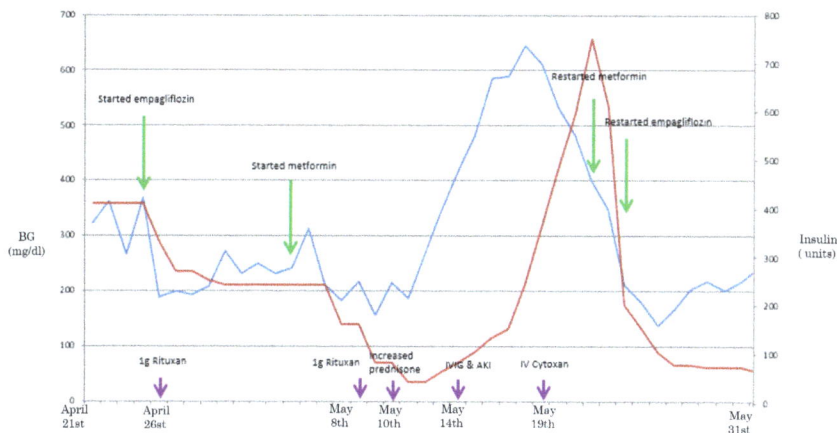

Figure 24.1—Blood glucose and insulin trend 1. IV, intravenous.

against the insulin receptor. Altered insulin signaling with subsequent severe insulin resistance results in uncontrolled diabetes. Refractory transient hyperglycemia, the most common presentation, occurs when high antibody titers exert an inhibitory effect on insulin receptors (insulin-resistant–like clinical picture). Paradoxically, hypoglycemia may rarely occur with activation of the insulin receptor in the setting of low antibody titers. TBIR is uncommon but the exact prevalence is unknown.[1] Typically, TBIR affects middle-aged African American females with an underlying autoimmune disorder such as autoimmune connective tissue disease, systemic lupus erythematosus (SLE), or thyroid, dermatologic, hematologic, or hepatic disease.[1]

Physicians should have a high index of suspicion for TBIR with this biochemical triad: elevated adiponectin level (>7 ng/mL), elevated fasting insulin

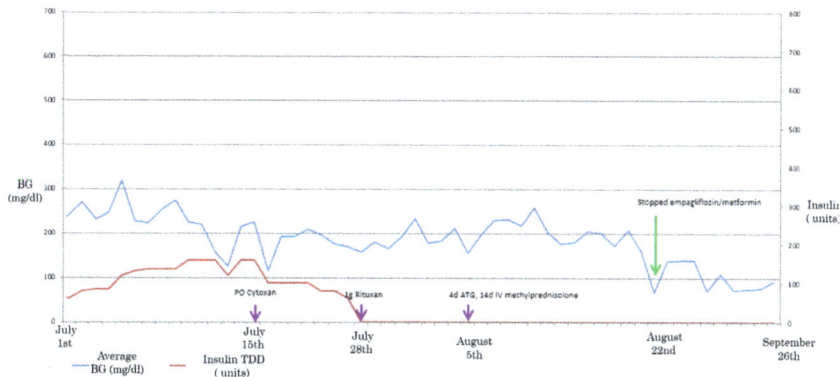

Figure 24.2—Blood glucose and insulin trend 2.

ANALYSIS FOR ANTI-INSR AUTO-ANTIBODIES: P1212

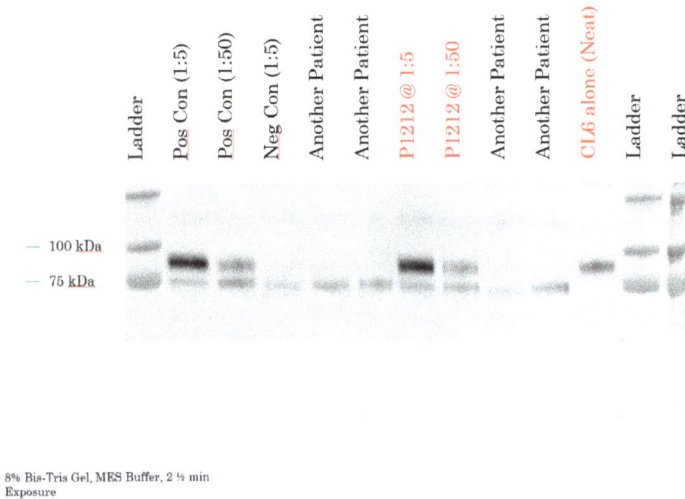

8% Bis-Tris Gel, MES Buffer, 2 ½ min Exposure

Figure 24.3—P1212 is positive for AIRAs at both concentrations tested.

concentration (>200 µIU/mL), and low/normal fasting triglyceride (TGs). Other clinical findings that should increase clinical suspicion include perioral/periocular acanthosis nigricans (AN) in nonobese individuals, hyperandrogenism, elevated HDL, hypercatabolism with unintentional weight loss (average of 43 ± 26 lb), and persistent hyperglycemia despite an insulin requirement of >3 units/kg/day. The presence of autoantibodies in the serum is confirmed by immunoprecipitation of recombinant human insulin receptors.[1]

The goal of treatment is to correct the metabolic derangements by controlling the production of autoantibodies using immunosuppressive therapy. Time to remission can vary from 2 to 9 months, with the average being 5 months.[1] We describe a case of TBIR initially treated with a sodium–glucose cotransporter 2 (SGLT2) inhibitor, with good response to the National Institutes of Health (NIH) protocol once the diagnosis was confirmed.

The classic manifestation of TBIR syndrome is severe hyperglycemia that is markedly resistant to high doses of insulin, or hypoglycemia.[1] AN, which is seen in 90% of patients with TBIR, develops abruptly along with symptomatic hyperglycemia. AN in TBIR frequently occurs over the perioral and periauricular areas. Other sites including the nape of the neck, axillae, groin, antecubital regions, popliteal fossae, and mucocutaneous surfaces of the lips and vulva may be involved. The proposed mechanism for this is the activation of one of three cellular receptors (epidermal growth factor receptor, fibroblast growth factor, and insulin-like growth factor).[1] As opposed to the more common forms of insulin resistance such as type 2 diabetes, where TG level is high and adiponectin is low, insulin resistance due to insulin receptor defects is paradoxically characterized by low TG and high adiponectin levels.[1] The hyperadiponectinemia resolves as the insulin receptor antibody concentration decreases.[2] Positive titers of AIRAs confirm the diagnosis, but this diagnosis is available only in research laboratories, since the serological test is not commercially available.[1]

Management of TBIR entails two forms of therapy: mitigation of glycemic abnormality and immune modulation. Initial measures should be aimed at alleviation of the catabolic state and prevention of further weight loss. To achieve this, extremely high doses of exogenous insulin via intravenous infusion followed by transitioning to U-500 concentrated regular insulin with close monitoring for hypoglycemia is necessary for the inpatient setting. AIRAs disrupt the receptor-mediated degradation of insulin, ultimately resulting in a prolonged half-life of insulin.[3] Other agents have been used for control of hyperglycemia in TBIR such as sulfonylureas, metformin, thiazolidinediones, and liraglutide. However, there have been conflicting results regarding the efficacy of these agents.[4] Before this report, there have not been cases in which SGLT2 inhibitor use has been published. These are promising results using a non–insulin-mediated mechanism to decrease insulin requirements. Hypoglycemia may be ameliorated by modification of the diet to involve meals at regular intervals, including a nighttime snack, to maintain blood glucose in the normal range. Glucocorticoids with doses equivalent to prednisone 20–150 mg are effective in reversing hypoglycemia. The effect is seen within 24 h of administration.[5]

Targeting the underlying autoimmune disorder guides the choice of immunomodulatory agents. The NIH protocol for the treatment of TBIR is composed of rituximab, monthly high-dose pulse glucocorticoids, and cyclophosphamide.[5] Rituximab is an antibody against CD-20, a cell surface molecule expressed by B-cell progenitors of antibody-producing cells and aimed at antibody-producing B lymphocytes. Pulse steroids were used to suppress the activity of preexisting antibody-producing plasma cells. Cyclophosphamide or cyclosporine (used in severe neutropenia) are used to amplify the suppression of both B- and T-cell function. The regimen should be switched to azathioprine at the onset of remission, defined as the amelioration of the hyperglycemia and discontinuation of insulin therapy. This therapeutic regimen was well tolerated with no serious adverse events in our patients.

In conclusion, TBIR is a rare disease with high mortality. Early diagnosis is important because it affects both the treatment and prognosis. With the use of appropriate immunosuppressive therapy, insulin resistance and metabolic abnormalities usually show significant improvement.

COMMENTARY

Type B insulin resistance is a rare autoimmune condition that nevertheless must be a part of the differential diagnosis in patients with severe insulin resistance, AN, hirsutism, and occasional hypoglycemia. It may occur in the context of other well-characterized autoimmune disorders such as lupus erythematosus or may suggest the presence of an autoimmune disease.

The onset of the disease is usually characterized by rapidly progressive nonketotic and severely insulin-resistant diabetes with paradoxical hypoglycemia. The diagnosis is based on the clinical picture and on detection of anti-insulin receptor autoantibodies in the serum, the hallmark of this syndrome. High doses of insulin are likely to be required to manage hyperinsulinemia, and occasional severe hypoglycemia is a dangerous complication of this condition. An interesting twist in this case is the use of SGLT2 inhibitors to manage hyperglycemia. The authors correctly stated that treatment of the underlying autoimmune disease is the cornerstone of management of TBIR. Prognosis depends on the underlying autoimmune disease, but unfortunately severe hypoglycemia may be fatal.

Boris Draznin, MD, PhD

REFERENCES

1. Arioglu E, Andewelt A, Diabo C, Bell M, Taylor SI, Gorden P. Clinical course of the syndrome of autoantibodies to the insulin receptor (type B insulin resistance): a 28-year perspective. *Medicine (Baltimore)* 2002;81:87–100

2. Semple RK, Halberg NH, Burling K, et al. Paradoxical elevation of high-molecular weight adiponectin in acquired extreme insulin resistance due to insulin receptor antibodies. *Diabetes* 2007;56:1712–1717

3. Cochran E, Musso C, Gorden P. The use of U-500 in patients with extreme insulin resistance. *Diabetes Care* 2005;28:1240–1244

4. Gehi A, Webb A, Nolte M, Davis J Jr. Treatment of systemic lupus erythematosus-associated type B insulin resistance syndrome with cyclophosphamide and mycophenolate mofetil. *Arthritis Rheum* 2003;48:1067–1070

5. Kang SM, Jin HY, Lee KA, Park JH, Baek HS, Park TS. Type B insulin-resistance syndrome presenting as autoimmune hypoglycemia, associated with systemic lupus erythematosus and interstitial lung disease. *Korean J Intern Med* 2013;28:98–102

Case 25

Latent Autoimmune Diabetes in an Adult With Insulin Allergy

Makeda Dawkins, MD,[1] and Alyson K. Myers, MD[2,3,4,5]

A 49-year-old African American female with a past medical history of hypothyroidism, psoriasis, and gestational diabetes (diet-controlled 20 years prior) was transferred from an outside hospital for an allergy consultation.

Two weeks prior, she went to a gynecologist for an annual exam. Her follow-up labs demonstrated an HbA$_{1c}$ of 8.8%. The patient was leaving for Cartagena, Columbia, the following day and was advised to exercise, decrease her carbohydrate intake, and see her primary care physician upon her return. On day 3 of her vacation, she developed nausea, decreased appetite, and emesis after meals. Her home fingerstick blood glucose was 500 mg/dL. She was sent to urgent care, where she was diagnosed with diabetic ketoacidosis (DKA) and treated with normal saline, potassium, and insulin infusions. During the transition to subcutaneous (SQ) insulin, she was given glargine insulin 15 units SQ and suddenly developed a bilateral arm rash. She was immediately treated with intravenous hydrocortisone 100 mg, improving her rash but elevating her blood glucose level.

The patient requested to be discharged and planned to continue treatment upon her return to the U.S. She was given another dose of glargine 15 units SQ, which caused subsequent lip swelling. She avoided carbohydrates during her flight home and immediately visited a local hospital upon landing. She was initially treated only with diphenhydramine and transferred to our facility for allergy consultation. Upon arrival, she had mild DKA, with an anion gap of 14, HCO$_3$ of 19 mmol/L, glucose of 315 mg/dL, and moderate ketones.

Past medical history: hypothyroidism
Past surgical history: none
Medications: Synthroid 75 μg p.o. daily (same dose for 5–6 years)
Allergies: dust, peaches, tree nuts, shellfish

[1]Department of Medicine, Westchester Medical Center, Valhalla, New York. [2]Department of Medicine, Division of Endocrinology, North Shore University Hospital, Northwell Health, Manhasset, New York. [3]Donald and Barbara Zucker School of Medicine at Hofstra/Northwell, Hempstead, New York. [4]Center for Health Innovations and Health Outcomes Research. [5]Feinstein Institute for Medical Research, Northwell Health, Manhasset, New York.

DOI: 10.2337/9781580407663.25

Social history: denies alcohol, tobacco, and illicit drug use
Family history: denies diabetes
Review of systems: positive for decreased appetite, nausea, vomiting, blurred vision, polyuria, polydipsia, neuropathy of hands bilaterally, arm rash bilaterally, and lip swelling

PHYSICAL EXAM

Vitals: temperature, 99.5°F; blood pressure, 119/77 mmHg; heart rate, 66 beats/min; respiration rate 11–25/min; oxygen saturation, 100% on room air; weight, 185 lb.

Exam unremarkable except for goiter with estimated size of 45 g.

HOSPITAL COURSE

This patient was presumed to have type 1 diabetes with an insulin analog allergy. Formal testing had to be deferred, since the patient had already received antihistamine therapy. Endocrinology and Allergy worked together to develop a regimen, beginning with an NPH and regular insulin challenge, with a goal of NPH 8 units b.i.d. SQ and regular insulin 4 units SQ three times daily (premeal) accompanied by a 1- to 3-unit correctional scale. The patient was observed in the intensive care unit with diphenhydramine 50 mg and an EpiPen at bedside. The challenge began with regular insulin 1 unit, followed by another 3 units 20 min later. Both doses were tolerated without hives, itching, swelling, angioedema, or respiratory or gastrointestinal symptoms. Two hours later, she was challenged with NPH 1 unit, followed by 3 units 20 min later, and the remaining 4 units 20 min following. This challenge was well tolerated, and she was discharged 2 days later with a regimen of NPH 10 units SQ twice a day and regular insulin 6 units SQ three times a day with meals.

FOLLOW-UP

During her ambulatory clinic follow-up, GAD65 and islet antigen 2 antibodies were found to be positive. Her C-peptide and serum glucose levels were 0.9 ng/mL and 349 mg/dL, respectively. She was maintained on NPH and regular insulin.

Allergic reactions in response to insulin analogs are rare, with an overall incidence of <1 to 2.4% in individuals with type 1 diabetes.[1] Local reactions can include swelling, erythema, and itching, with the possibility of generalizing to angioedema and eventually anaphylaxis. Allergic reactions to glargine are less common than reactions in response to detemir and other insulins, warranting the use of glargine as an alternative for patients with established allergies.[1] Glargine is a slowly metabolized long-acting insulin, rarely inducing immediate immune responses, and is commonly formulated with zinc and/or metacresol to delay absorption.[1] Patients can be allergic to the glargine monomers themselves or zinc or metacresol allergens, highlighting the need for specific intradermal as well as IgG and IgE testing.

Regardless of the etiology, first-line management for assumed or established insulin allergy includes symptomatic relief with antihistamines and switching insulin preparations or transitioning to oral agents in the case of type 2 diabetes. More severe allergic reactions may be treated with combinations of antihistamines in addition to a histamine 2 antagonist and systemic steroids.[1] Airway patency should be continually assessed and maintained. One method to induce tolerance is through the use of continuous subcutaneous insulin infusion via pump therapy, starting at very low and progressively increasing basal dosages.[2] Tolerance may also be established via desensitization, using immunotherapy with progressive insulin administration.[3] This approach is hypothesized to act via the induction of T-regulatory cells, depletion of specific T-cells, and mediation of antibody production by cytokines.[3]

Although immediate hypersensitivity to insulin analogs is increasingly rare among patients with latent autoimmune diabetes in adults (LADA), management recommendations still reflect those of any other drug intolerance. Intra-dermal and antibody testing should be performed while another insulin preparation is administered and observed for tolerance. In this case, the testing was deferred since the patient had already been treated with antihistamine therapy.

COMMENTARY

Allergic reactions to insulin have been described from the time insulin was discovered. Allergy to insulin analogs, however, are very rare, and allergic reactions to glargine are exceedingly rare. However, cases of allergy to insulin analogs continue to be reported. Allergic reactions can be localized and affect a specific area or systemic. The latter are usually due to the insulin molecule itself rather than additives and/or preservatives. The reactions can be immediate, intermediate (30 min to 6 h after insulin injection), or delayed (usually with insulin containing zinc).

The authors describe meticulous attention to her allergy and excellent treatment approach. The case, however, also indicates that going on vacation 1 day after diabetes is diagnosed is probably not prudent. Luckily, she survived both DKA in a foreign country and an insulin allergy.

Boris Draznin, MD, PhD

REFERENCES

1. Badik J, Chen J, Letvak K, So TY. Hypersensitivity reaction to insulin glargine and insulin detemir in a pediatric patient: a case report. *J Pediatr Pharmacol Ther* 2016;21:85–91. doi:10.5863/1551-6776-21.1.85

2. Hasselmann C, Pecquet C, Bismuth E, et al. Continuous subcutaneous insulin infusion allows tolerance induction and diabetes treatment in a type 1 diabetic child with insulin allergy. *Diabetes Metab* 2013;39:174–117

3. Jutel M, Akdis M, Budak F. IL-10 and TGF-beta cooperate in the regulatory T cell response to mucosal allergens in normal immunity and specific immunotherapy. *Eur J Immunol* 2003;33:1205–1214

Case 26

Onset of Autoimmune Diabetes During Pregnancy

Kaitlyn Barrett, DO,[1] Kelsey Sheahan, MD,[1] and
Matthew P. Gilbert, DO, MPH[1]

A 30-year-old G4P3 female was referred for evaluation of diabetes during her third trimester of pregnancy. Her pre-pregnancy BMI was 22 kg/m². She did not have a history of gestational diabetes during her three preceding pregnancies. Her largest newborn weighed 8 lb, 6 oz, at birth. During her routine oral glucose tolerance test (OGTT), her blood glucose level was 260 mg/dL 1 h after a 50-g oral glucose load, diagnostic of diabetes. Subsequent laboratory studies revealed a positive GAD antibody of 0.1 nmol/L (reference ≤0.02 nmol/L), C-peptide of 3.5 ng/mL (reference range 1.1–4.4 ng/mL), and HbA$_{1c}$ of 5.8% (reference range 4.0–5.6%). She had a family history of type 1 diabetes in her sister.

Hyperglycemia during pregnancy is characterized by adverse birth complications including macrosomia and preeclampsia. As such, the American Diabetes Association (ADA) recommends that all pregnant patients are routinely screened for gestational diabetes during the second trimester (24–28 weeks of gestation) with an OGTT.[1] Gestational diabetes has routinely been defined as diabetes with the first recognition during the second or third trimester pregnancy.[1,2] It is estimated, however, that 6% of patients with gestational diabetes are autoantibody positive.[2] Currently, guidelines do not recommend screening for autoantibodies during pregnancy. However, screening for diabetes in reproductive age females is not widely performed; therefore, gestational diabetes may represent preexisting diabetes that has not otherwise been diagnosed.

The ADA recommends the same glycemic targets for women with type 1 and type 2 diabetes during pregnancy: fasting glucose <95 mg/dL, 1-h postprandial glucose <140 mg/dL, and 2-h postprandial glucose <120 mg/dL.[3]

Because of the degree of hyperglycemia, medical nutrition therapy alone was not attempted in this patient. She was started on long-acting insulin with glargine, which was titrated to a fasting blood glucose goal of <95 mg/dL, and she was referred to Endocrinology. At the time of her Endocrinology visit, she was taking glargine 25 units daily and lispro 13 units with meals

---

[1]Department of Medicine, Division of Endocrinology and Diabetes, Larner College of Medicine at The University of Vermont, Burlington, Vermont.

DOI: 10.2337/9781580407663.26

and working with a nutritionist to monitor carbohydrate intake. At the visit, she reported fasting blood glucose levels of 75–100 mg/dL, 2-h postprandial glucose levels from breakfast and lunch of 100–140 mg/dL, and 2-h postprandial levels from dinner of 75–110 mg/dL. While these levels are acceptable, she also reported nocturnal hypoglycemia, and so her glargine dose was reduced.

The patient had an uncomplicated vaginal delivery at 38 weeks. She was monitored for hyperglycemia immediately postpartum with routine blood glucose testing. She did not require any insulin postpartum and was discharged with instructions to monitor her blood glucose off all insulin.

There is a dramatic reduction in insulin resistance immediately postpartum.[3] As gestational diabetes may represent previously undiagnosed type 2 diabetes, or in this case, antibody-positive diabetes, screening and continued evaluation in the postpartum period is critical. The HbA$_{1c}$ may still be affected by increased red blood cell turnover during pregnancy; therefore, the ADA recommends performing an OGTT at 4–12 weeks postpartum. In addition, because of the lifetime risk for diabetes associated with gestational diabetes, women with a history of gestational diabetes should have ongoing screening indefinitely.[3]

She returned to the Endocrinology clinic 4 months later. Sporadic at-home blood glucose testing revealed values ranging from 60 to 140 mg/dL. Point-of-care HbA$_{1c}$ was measured to be 5.5%. A 1-h OGTT was not performed because it was felt that it would not change management. Education was provided surrounding signs and symptoms of overt diabetes and the possibility of developing type 1 diabetes.

Women who test positive for antibodies should be counseled about the risk of developing diabetes, including the symptoms of diabetes and prevention of diabetic ketoacidosis (DKA). In addition, it is recommended that women with gestational diabetes be tested at 4–12 weeks postpartum, using a 75-g OGTT and other appropriate non-pregnancy diagnostic criteria such as HbA$_{1c}$.[3]

At her next follow-up Endocrinology appointment 3 months later (6 months postpartum), her HbA$_{1c}$ was 5.8%. She was not started on any medications but counseled again on the signs and symptoms of diabetes and DKA with a plan to recheck her HbA$_{1c}$ in 6 months.

Patients who are found to have islet autoantibodies during pregnancy are at a high risk of progression to overt type 1 diabetes after delivery.[2] As shown in Figure 26.1, the presence of autoantibodies has been found to correlate with an earlier insulin requirement.[5] This condition has been compared to latent autoimmune diabetes in adults (LADA) because of the variation in the degree of progression. This patient's presentation, including the lack of overt symptoms and ketosis after pregnancy and adult-onset and positive antibodies, is consistent with LADA.[4]

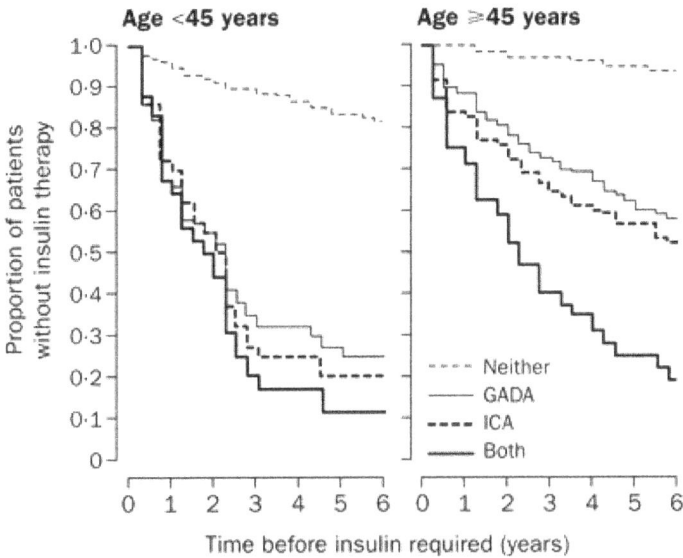

Figure 26.1 — Patients with and without islet cell cytoplasmic autoantibodies (ICAs) and GAD autoantibodies (GADA) requiring insulin therapy during 6 years of follow-up.[4]

COMMENTARY

This is an interesting case of gestational diabetes in a woman with positive GAD antibody, normal C-peptide, and HbA$_{1c}$ in the prediabetes range (5.8%). She was treated with insulin, had an uncomplicated vaginal delivery, and remained off insulin at 6 months postpartum. She is not "out of the woods" yet, and it would be interesting to see the titer of other autoantibodies, as the positivity in more than one would greatly increase her risk for developing type 1 diabetes. As the authors correctly point out, if she were to have late autoimmune diabetes of adulthood, despite more mild initial course of diabetes, she would require insulin therapy sooner rather than later. Thus, close follow up is the key to timely diagnosis and treatment.

Boris Draznin, MD, PhD

REFERENCES

1. American Diabetes Association. 2. Classification and diagnosis of diabetes: *Standards of Medical Care in Diabetes—2020*. *Diabetes Care* 2020;43(Suppl. 1):S14–S31

2. Nilsson C, Ursing D, Törn C, Aberg A, Landin-Olsson M. Presence of GAD antibodies during gestational diabetes mellitus predicts type 1 diabetes. *Diabetes Care* 2007;30:1968–1971

3. American Diabetes Association. 14. Management of diabetes in pregnancy: *Standards of Medical Care in Diabetes—2020. Diabetes Care* 2020;43(Suppl. 1): S183–S192

4. Dunn JP, Perkins JM, Jagasia SM. Latent autoimmune diabetes in adults and pregnancy: foretelling the future. *Clinical Diabetes* 2008;26:44–46

5. Turner R, Stratton I, Horton V, et al. UKPDS25: autoantibodies to islet-cell cytoplasm and glutamic acid decarboxylase for prediction of insulin requirement in type 2 diabetes. *Lancet* 1997:350:1288–1293

Case 27

Comorbidity of Diabetes and Systemic Lupus Erythematosus

Boris Mankovsky, MD,[1,2] and Yanina Saenko, MD[2]

Patient N.V., a 57-year-old Caucasian female, was admitted to our hospital with chief complaints of newly developed skin lesions on the face and thorax that appeared a few weeks prior, as well high glucose levels, thirst, and polyuria.

The patient was diagnosed with diabetes in 2007 (13 years ago) when she presented with thirst, weight loss (6.6 lb), polyuria, fatigue, itching, and high glucose levels (>15 mmol/L or 270 mg/dL). The diagnosis of type 2 diabetes was made, and the patient was treated with metformin for the next 5 years. Normoglycemia was never achieved, and HbA_{1c} levels fluctuated around 9% at all times. In 2012, she was started on insulin glargine, once daily in addition to metformin. During the following years, HbA_{1c} decreased but remained around 8% despite an increase in the dose of glargine and introduction of mealtime insulin glulisine. The patient's C-peptide was at the lower limit of the reference range (1.08 ng/mL), and GAD antibodies were negative.

Her medical history was remarkable for arterial hypertension, dyslipidemia, and continuous decline of glomerular filtration rate, decreasing from 52 mL/min in 2014 to 40 mL/min in 2020. She also had autoimmune thyroiditis without significant elevation of thyroid-stimulating hormone (TSH) levels (around 5–6 µIU/L since first detected). She was taking appropriate antihypertensive medications and a statin.

During the current admission, the patient was examined by Dermatology and Rheumatology. Skin biopsy was performed, which revealed changes highly suggestive of the subacute phase of systemic lupus erythematosus. Laboratory findings including significantly elevated erythrocyte sedimentation rate and C-reactive protein, along with increased levels of antinuclear antibodies, were consistent with the diagnosis of systemic lupus erythematosus, and treatment with glucocorticoid was initiated.

The patient has three diseases that occurred simultaneously: diabetes, autoimmune thyroiditis, and systemic lupus erythematosus. We believe that this case illustrates the increased risk of the comorbidity of different autoimmune

[1]Department of Diabetology, National Medical Academy for Postgraduate Education.
[2]Center for Innovative Medical Technologies, Kiev, Ukraine.
DOI: 10.2337/9781580407663.27

diseases with diabetes. On the other hand, the diagnosis of systemic lupus erythematosus prompted us to reconsider the initial diagnosis of type 2 diabetes.

The patient was diagnosed with type 2 diabetes at the time of initial diabetes diagnosis. However, it is notable that oral hypoglycemic treatment never resulted in good metabolic control, and insulin had to be prescribed quite early in the course of disease. Moreover, apparently, intensive insulin treatment with multiple daily injections of short- and long-acting insulins was required to control her glycemia. C-peptide level at the time of the current examination was found to be quite low relative to simultaneous plasma glucose levels, which were in the high range. This low level of insulin production at the current time can be attributed to the longstanding duration of diabetes (>10 years), but one can speculate that insulin production may have been quite low on initial presentation of diabetes. These points suggest reconsideration of the diagnosis of diabetes as type 1 diabetes or latent autoimmune diabetes in adults (LADA). Because anti-GAD antibodies were not elevated, such a diagnosis could not be confirmed. However, it is possible that elevated anti-GAD antibody levels might have been present at the time of onset, but disappeared subsequently, 13 years after the onset of diabetes.

The suspected diagnosis of type 1 diabetes in this patient is based on the well-known and documented association of this type of diabetes with other autoimmune diseases.

Recently, one of the largest studies in this area, the Finnish Nationwide Study, found that almost every fifth patient (22.8%) with type 1 diabetes also had another autoimmune disease, with more females than males having such an association—31.6 and 14.9%, respectively.[1] Autoimmune diseases associated with type 1 diabetes included hypothyroidism, hyperthyroidism, celiac disease, Addison's disease, and atrophic gastritis. Late onset of type 1 diabetes and aging increase the risk of hypothyroidism. Clinical features presented in this case (an onset of diabetes at age 44 years and an association with autoimmune thyroiditis) seem to be in agreement with the results of this study. In a recent meta-analysis of studies totaling >290,000 patients with type 1 diabetes, the association of diabetes with autoimmune diseases such as celiac disease, gastric autoimmunity including pernicious anemia, vitiligo, and adrenal insufficiency was confirmed, while hypothyroidism and celiac disease were the most frequently found.[2]

Systemic lupus erythematosus is associated with an increased risk of developing an endocrine disease. However, the association of lupus with diabetes is not well characterized. In a recent retrospective analysis of a cohort of more than 700 patients with systemic lupus erythematosus, the most common endocrinopathy was hypothyroidism (5.22%) followed by type 2 diabetes (1.41%) and hyperthyroidism (1.41%), type 1 diabetes (0.42%), and hyperparathyroidism (0.70%).[3] Contrary to our case, the diagnosis of systemic lupus erythematosus preceded the development of endocrinopathies, while in our patient the diagnosis of diabetes was made long before the onset of symptoms of systemic lupus erythematosus. It is of interest that 21.8% of patients with systemic lupus erythematosus and other endocrine disease have an increased risk of developing a second endocrine disease, similar to the case presented herein, with three endocrine diseases affecting the same patient.

We have to admit that because systemic lupus erythematosus can be associated with both type 1 and type 2 diabetes, the mere association cannot allow re-classification of diabetes type. The patient is now treated with multiple injections of insulin for her glycemic control, making the precise diagnosis of type of diabetes more of an academic exercise without practical implications. We believe that this clinical case underscores the importance of the association of diabetes with other autoimmune diseases, including systemic lupus erythematosus, and should be well recognized by physicians.

COMMENTARY

This case brings to light a few interesting points. The first is that diabetes is associated with other autoimmune diseases, both endocrine and non-endocrine in nature. While association of endocrine autoimmune diseases with diabetes is well known, an association with non-endocrine conditions has received much less attention. The second interesting point is that systemic lupus erythematosus can be associated with both types of diabetes. Based on what we know about this particular case, it is more likely that the patient has type 2 diabetes. However, as the authors have correctly pointed out, because the patient is treated with multiple daily insulin injections, the importance of classification is more academic than practical. Finally, timely initiation of insulin therapy in patients with poorly controlled diabetes is critical for prevention of acute and chronic complications of diabetes and is worthy of additional emphasis.

Boris Draznin, MD, PhD

REFERENCES

1. Mäkimattila S, Harjutsalo V, Forsblom C, Groop P-H, on behalf of the FinnDiane Study Group. Every fifth individual with type 1 diabetes suffers from an additional autoimmune disease: a Finnish nationwide study. *Diabetes Care* 2020;43:1041–1047

2. Nederstigt C, Uitbeijerse BS, Janssen LGM, Corssmit EPM, de Koning EJP, Dekkers OM. Associated auto-immune disease in type 1 diabetes patients: a systematic review and meta-analysis. *Eur J Endocrinol* 2019;180:135–144

3. Muñoz C, Isenberg DA. Review of major endocrine abnormalities in patients with systemic lupus erythematosus. *Clin Exp Rheumatol* 2019;37:791–796

Case 28

Illusion of Autoimmune Diabetes

Nay Linn Aung, MD[1]

A 62-year-old Caucasian woman with a history of hypertension was diagnosed with type 2 diabetes at the age of 56 years during a routine medical checkup. She was started on metformin, and later empagliflozin and glipizide were added. However, the patient stopped taking metformin because of gastrointestinal side effects after a few months. HbA_{1c} over time is shown in Table 28.1.

She had a family history of diabetes in both of her parents, her nephew, and three cousins. Her nephew had been treated with insulin. The patient had a normal BMI ranging from 21–25 kg/m². She denied taking steroids or any medication that might cause hyperglycemia. She denied a history of obstructive sleep apnea. She reported drinking socially and smoking about one pack of cigarettes a day. The patient denied any history of diabetic ketoacidosis (DKA), and frequent or severe hypoglycemia. She had no known micro- or macrovascular complications. Her blood pressure had been well controlled with losartan 50 mg daily. On exam, the patient did not have central adiposity, acanthosis nigricans, or skin tags.

Her lipid panel showed the following result: triglycerides 119 mg/dL; total cholesterol 192 mg/dL; LDL 80.2 mg/dL; and HDL 88 mg/dL. C-peptide ordered by her primary care provider just before the referral was 2.4 ng/mL, with random blood glucose of 397 mg/dL.

At her initial visit, low-dose extended-release metformin was resumed and liraglutide was added. The patient's HbA_{1c} improved to 8.6%; however, it was not sustained and increased to 9.6% within 6 months. Because of failure to improve blood glucose control on four different antidiabetic medications, and the lack of signs consistent with insulin resistance, C-peptide and autoantibodies were ordered (Table 28.2).

After reviewing these labs, glipizide, empagliflozin, and liraglutide were discontinued and basal insulin plus mealtime insulin at the largest meal were initiated. The patient gained about 17 lb within 3 months of starting insulin therapy, which interfered with her adherence to insulin, since this

[1]St. Elizabeth Family Medicine Residency, Mohawk Valley Health System (MVHS), Utica, New York.

DOI: 10.2337/9781580407663.28

Table 28.1 — HbA$_{1c}$ over time

	2/25/2015	6/18/2015	9/14/2015	03/15/2016	10/14/2016	4/10/2017
HbA$_{1c}$ (%)	9.2	8.3	6.4	6.2	6.7	7.1
	8/28/2017	1/24/2018	5/2/2018	7/23/2018	12/31/2018	6/7/2019
	7.3	8.5	8.4	7.8	9.9	9.6

weight gain was unwanted. A glucagon-like peptide (GLP)-1 receptor agonist was restarted to counteract weight gain as well as for glycemic control. The patient's self-reported blood glucose has improved since then.

Correct classification of diabetes is important for instituting appropriate treatment and reducing therapeutic inertia in people with diabetes. To classify diabetes correctly solely based on phenotypic observation can be challenging. Some patients initially diagnosed with type 2 diabetes can have positive autoantibodies, especially in individuals who are younger at diagnosis.[1,2]

The etiology and pathogenesis of type 2 diabetes is not fully understood. However, peripheral insulin resistance (IR) with lack of autoimmune destruction of β-cells are major features of the pathogenesis of type 2 diabetes. Central adiposity (with or without obesity or overweight), smoking, and obstructive sleep apnea are associated strongly with IR. Steroids and other medications are also linked to IR and play a role in drug-induced diabetes.[3] Acanthosis nigricans and skin tags may be seen in people with IR.

Latent autoimmune diabetes in adults (LADA) is a form of slow progression of immune-mediated diabetes. Autoimmune markers including islet cell autoantibodies and autoantibodies to GAD (GAD65), insulin, the tyrosine phosphatases IA-2 and IA-2β, and zinc transporter 8 (ZnT8) are associated with LADA. The rate of β-cell destruction may vary, especially in patients with LADA. These patients may retain β-cell function at the early stage, but there is little or no insulin secretion at the later stage, which is manifest by low or undetectable plasma C-peptide. It is recommended that adults without traditional risk factors and young adults who are newly diagnosed with diabetes undergo autoantibody testing.[3]

Table 28.2 — C-peptide and antibody levels

Random blood glucose	172 mg/dL
C-peptide (reference 1.1–4.4 ng/mL)	1.8
GAD65 antibodies (reference ≤0.02 nmol/L)	48.2
IA-2 antibodies (reference ≤0.02 nmol/L)	1.33

IA, protein tyrosine phosphatase.

Our patient lacked features and risk factors for IR, except smoking. Therefore, C-peptide was ordered by her primary care provider. C-peptide along with GAD65 and IA-2A antibodies were ordered again in our clinic 6 months later. Both times, her C-peptide was within the normal range; however, GAD65 and IA-2A were significantly elevated. Because C-peptide levels can be normal in the early stages, LADA diagnosis should not be ruled out solely based on normal C-peptide. Although the patient may have insulin reserve at this time, individuals with positive antibodies can develop significant hyperglycemia and even DKA quickly, especially during stress and infection.[3]

Available randomized clinical trials do not support a specific treatment algorithm for patients with LADA. Because LADA manifests itself in different clinical phenotypes, successful treatment of diabetes in these patients requires a personalized approach with careful attention to the timing of conversion to insulin therapy. Reviews of potential pharmacological approaches to LADA can be found in the recent publications by Buzzetti et al.[4] and Brophy et al.[5] The overall consensus is that most patients with LADA require insulin therapy much earlier than patients with type 2 diabetes.

COMMENTARY

This is an interesting, rare, but not totally unusual case presentation of a patient with probable LADA. The American Diabetes Association does not recognize LADA as a distinct entity and includes LADA within the type 1 diabetes classification in the spectrum of phenotypic presentations of autoimmune diabetes. The important point of this case and of many other cases of LADA is to keep this diagnosis in mind while attending to patients with diabetes who present therapeutic challenges. Proper and timely identification of the autoimmune process leads to timely initiation of insulin therapy, which is critical. For now, insulin therapy remains the cornerstone of successful glycemic control in these patients.

Boris Draznin, MD, PhD

REFERENCES

1. Davis TME, Wright AD, Mehta ZM, et al. Islet autoantibodies in clinically diagnosed type 2 diabetes: prevalence and relationship with metabolic control (UKPDS 70). *Diabetologia* 2005;48:695–702

2. Zinman B, Kahn SE, Haffner SM, et al. Phenotypic characteristics of GAD antibody-positive recently diagnosed patients with type 2 diabetes in North America and Europe. *Diabetes* 2004;53:3193–3200

3. American Diabetes Association. 2. Classification and diagnosis of diabetes: *Standards of Medical Care in Diabetes—2020. Diabetes Care* 2020;43(Suppl. 1): S14–S31

4. Buzzetti R, Zampetti S, Maddaloni E. Adult-onset autoimmune diabetes: current knowledge and implications for management. *Nat Rev Endocrinol* 2017;13:674–686

5. Brophy S, Davies H, Mannan S, Brunt H, Williams R. Interventions for latent autoimmune diabetes (LADA) in adults. *Cochrane Database Syst Rev* 2011:CD006165

Can a Lupus Flare Cause Autoimmune Diabetes?

Andriy Havrylyan, MD[1], and Janice L. Gilden, MS, MD[1,2]

A 62-year-old female with systemic lupus erythematosus (SLE) diagnosed in 1997, with renal biopsy confirming nephritis and later pulmonary involvement, autoimmune hypothyroidism, autoimmune hemolytic anemia, Raynaud's phenomenon, myasthenia gravis, and fibromyalgia, was referred to Endocrinology for worsening hyperglycemia during acute hospitalization for shortness of breath. The patient had previously been diagnosed with type 2 diabetes treated with metformin. She was taking prednisone chronically at varying doses (5 mg b.i.d. to 60 mg daily) depending on SLE disease activity. The blood glucose levels significantly increased when the steroid dose was increased because of lupus pneumonitis, and she subsequently developed autoimmune hemolytic anemia with hemoglobin level dropping from 12.7 g/dL (normal range 12.0–16.0) to 5.8 g/dL. HbA_{1c} had increased from 5.7 to 8.0%, with blood glucose values upwards of 400 mg/dL while hospitalized. It was assumed that insulin resistance had worsened, because of high steroid doses of methylprednisolone 125 mg every 8 h. She was started on basal-bolus insulin therapy. The patient was also treated with one dose of intravenous immunoglobulin preparation 1 g/kg for immune-mediated hemolytic anemia. Although previously negative, GAD65 antibodies became positive, suggesting autoimmune diabetes. She also had islet antibodies measured during that time, but results were nonspecific, and the laboratory could not rule out the presence of islet antibodies.

In subsequent months, she was taken off insulin therapy, since she was weaned off of her steroid dose. Two years later, the patient developed overnight hypoglycemia, as confirmed by a continuous glucose monitoring device, while off all antidiabetic agents, without any change in her weight or BMI of 28 kg/m². An ACTH stimulation test showed adequate adrenal function with adrenal antibodies remaining negative. She had a repeat blood test for GAD65 and islet antibodies, which had now become negative (Table 29.1).

It has been described in the literature that patients with one autoimmune condition have a higher risk for developing other autoimmune conditions.

[1]Diabetes/Endocrinology Section, Chicago Medical School at Rosalind Franklin University of Medicine and Science. [2]Captain James A. Lovell Federal Health Care Center, North Chicago, Illinois.

 DOI: 10.2337/9781580407663.29

Table 29.1—Laboratory data

Time	GAD65 antibodies (IU/mL)	Islet cell antibody	HbA$_{1c}$ (reference 4.0–6.0)	CRP (reference 0.0–0.9)	Intravenous immunoglobulin
+11 months	<5	Negative	5.8%	<0.3	
+10 months		Negative			
+8 months			6.3%		
+10 days	117	Cannot rule out presence			
+1 days				5.1	1 g/kg
0	Acute hospitalization for SLE with high-dose steroid therapy				
−5 days	<5		8.0%	3.4	
−5 months			5.7%	<0.3	
−9 months			5.5%		

Autoimmune polyendocrine syndromes (APSs) are types of endocrine organ dysfunction caused by autoimmunity. They can stem from genetic susceptibility as well as loss of immune tolerance. The more common variant of APS is type 2 (APS-2), characterized by at least two of the following three autoimmune conditions: type 1 diabetes, autoimmune thyroiditis, and primary adrenal insufficiency. APS-2 is polygenic, affects more women than men, usually presents in adulthood, and results from loss of immune tolerance, in which T-cells become autoreactive with resulting lymphocytic infiltration and dysfunction of affected tissues and organs. Circulating autoantibodies can confirm the diagnosis. APS-2 has been described in association with other autoimmune conditions (celiac disease, primary ovarian insufficiency, SLE, rheumatoid arthritis, vitiligo, alopecia, myasthenia gravis, and autoimmune gastritis).

Physicians often rely on serological testing for autoantibodies to either screen high-risk patients or to confirm a diagnosis in a patient with clinical symptoms. The drawback is that patients develop autoimmunity over time and a single negative serological test does not ensure that the patient will not develop disease in the future. Testing for autoantibodies in type 1 diabetes includes islet cell antibodies (ICAs), insulin autoantibodies (IAAs), tyrosine phosphatase (IA-2), zinc transporter 8 (ZnT8s), and most commonly GAD65.

GAD is the major enzyme in the synthesis of γ-aminobutyric acid (GABA), which functions as an inhibitory neurotransmitter. There are two isoforms of GAD (GAD65 and GAD67), with GAD65 present in pancreatic tissue and both isoforms present in neuronal tissue. High GAD antibody titers have been shown to be present in neurologic diseases such as stiff person syndrome, cerebellar ataxia, limbic encephalitis, and epilepsy, but the association is unclear.[1]

GAD65 is arguably the most commonly tested autoantibody in testing for type 1 diabetes with sensitivity, specificity, positive predictive values, and negative predictive values of 60.8, 100.0, 100.0, and 71.8% by enzyme-linked immunosorbent assay (ELISA).[2] It has been documented that 1.7% of individuals who tested positive for anti-GAD were persistently nondiabetic, and about 53.9% converting to anti-GAD–negative serology in an approximately 10-year span.[3] There is also data in the literature showing that individuals with higher GAD antibody titers have higher progression to insulin deficiency.[4]

Herein, we describe a case of a woman with multiple autoimmune disorders and the presence of fluctuating antibodies to GAD65 and islet cells during increased disease activity of SLE. Our patient developed transient elevation of GAD65 antibodies during an acute episode of SLE. Acute hyperglycemia during hospitalization can largely be attributed to high doses of steroids. However, the significance of an increased HbA_{1c} level of 8.0% shortly before hospitalization and prior to high steroid treatment is not clear. A seroconversion of GAD65 antibodies was observed during increased rheumatologic disease activity with its associated surge in cytokines and chemokines, suggesting a possible association. Another possible explanation for GAD65 seroconversion is that the patient was receiving therapy with intravenous immunoglobulin (IV Ig), which may cause false-positive ELISA testing for GAD antibodies. Most commercially available IV Ig preparations contain anti-GAD antibodies measurable by ELISA testing in titers ranging from 40 to 1,507 IU/mL.[5] Diagnostic testing of GAD antibodies in patients after IV Ig therapy can lead to false-positive results and misdiagnosis.

COMMENTARY

Even though SLE is frequently associated with other autoimmune conditions, including type 1 diabetes, its association with type 2 diabetes is not uncommon. Worsening of glycemic control can be a consequence of increased insulin resistance induced by SLE in and of itself or, more commonly, be a result of steroid therapy. In this case, both a flare of SLE and initiation of high steroid treatment could explain deterioration of glycemic control in this patient. An unusual feature of this case is transient elevations in anti-GAD antibody titer during the SLE flare. The cause and even the authenticity of GAD65 seroconversion remain enigmatic, as the authors carefully and thoughtfully discuss. Clinically, however, it is important to keep in mind that glycemic control can be negatively affected by SLE activity and treatment.

Boris Draznin, MD, PhD

REFERENCES

1. Nakajima H, Nakamura Y, Inaba Y, et al. Neurologic disorders associated with anti-glutamic acid decarboxylase antibodies: a comparison of anti-GAD antibody titers and time-dependent changes between neurologic disease and type I diabetes mellitus. *J Neuroimmunol* 2018;317:84–89. doi: 10.1016/j.jneuroim.2018.01.007

2. Murata T, Tsuzaki K, Nirengi S, et al. Diagnostic accuracy of the anti-glutamic acid decarboxylase antibody in type 1 diabetes mellitus: comparison between radioimmunoassay and enzyme-linked immunosorbent assay. *J Diabetes Investig* 2017;8:475–479. doi: 10.1111/jdi.12594

3. Sorgjerd EP, Thorsby PM, Torjesen PA et al. Presence of anti-GAD is a non-diabetic population of adults: time dynamics and clinical influence: results from the HUNT study. *BMJ Open Diabetes Res Care* 2015;3:e000076. doi: 10.1136/bmjdrc-2014-000076

4. Lee SA, Lee WJ, Kim EH, et al. Progression to insulin deficiency in Korean patients with type 2 diabetes mellitus positive for anti-GAD antibody. *Diabet Med* 2011;28:319–324. doi: 10.1111/j.1464-5491.2010.03186.x

5. Dimitriadou MM, Alexopoulos H, Akrivou S, et al. Anti-neuronal antibodies within the IVIg preparations: importance in clinical practice. *Neurotherapeutics* 2020;17:235–242. https://doi.org/10.1007/s13311-019-00796-3

Part 5

Continuous Glucose Monitoring (CGM) and Insulin Pumps

Case 30

Feasibility and Utility of Continuous Glucose Monitoring in an Adult With Type 1 Diabetes and Down's Syndrome

Kristen L. Flint, MD,[1] and Elena Toschi, MD[1,2]

A 30-year-old male with Down's syndrome, type 1 diabetes, and hypothyroidism presented to the adult endocrinology clinic with his father. His history was significant for type 1 diabetes, diagnosed at 2 years of age, complicated by mild nonproliferative diabetic retinopathy and the inability to communicate symptoms of hypoglycemia. He was on multiple daily injection (MDI) therapy of insulin: NPH 30 units plus rapid-acting insulin scale QAM before breakfast, and NPH 9 units plus rapid-acting scale QPM before dinner. He was on 50 µg levothyroxine daily. His laboratory data included HbA$_{1c}$ of 8.1%, undetectable C-peptide (<0.01 ng/mL), and thyroid-stimulating hormone (TSH) of 2.5 µIU/L.

He lives with his father and stepmother, who share responsibilities over his daily activities and health care, including administration of his medications. He has a consistent schedule and food intake. He wakes at 7:00 A.M., eats breakfast, and his father administers morning NPH and rapid-acting insulin as per plan. He goes to daycare from 8:00 A.M. to 1:30 P.M., where his caregivers give him frequent snacks to prevent potential hypoglycemic episodes. However, they do not administer insulin for hyperglycemia. He eats lunch around noon and has another snack in the afternoon. After daycare, he is home alone until 3:30 P.M. when his parents return. He eats dinner around 6:00 P.M., at which time his blood glucose is checked, and evening NPH and rapid-acting insulin are given as per plan.

Review of self-monitored blood glucose revealed high glucose variability throughout the day: fasting morning glucose of 45–339 mg/dL, lunchtime glucose of 65–326 mg/dL, and a similar dinnertime glucose range but with fewer episodes of hypoglycemia. Notably, the patient is unable to express symptoms of hypoglycemia, and caregivers worry about his hypoglycemic episodes and their complications.

At first visit, it was decided to start him on personal continuous glucose monitoring (CGM). His caregivers were instructed how to insert and use CGM. He continued on the same daily routine. On follow-up, CGM showed time spent in hypoglycemia (<70 mg/dL) of 7% (~100 min/day), with hypoglycemic episodes occurring mostly overnight (Table 30.1). Therefore, his

[1]Department of Medicine, Beth Israel Deaconess Medical Center, Boston, Massachusetts.
[2]Joslin Diabetes Center, Boston, Massachusetts.

DOI: 10.2337/9781580407663.30

evening NPH was reduced to 7 units. His father was taught to monitor and adjust his insulin depending on glucose level, physical activity, and food intake. His daycare caregivers could also access the data and adjust snacks accordingly.

At his 6-month follow-up visit, he showed improvement with the new insulin regimen and increased attention to diabetes care by caregivers. His average glucose increased to 169 mg/dL, but time in range (TIR 70–180 mg/dL) increased from 49% to 58% (~130 min/day), and he had markedly less time below range (TBR <70 mg/dL), from 7% to 1% (reduction of 86 min/day). Glucose variability assessed by the coefficient of variation (CV) improved (Table 30.1). His HbA_{1c} improved to 7.5%.

Individuals with Down's syndrome have a 4.2-fold greater prevalence of type 1 diabetes compared to the general pediatric population.[1] Certain genetic components on chromosome 21 may confer increased risk of type 1 diabetes, but the mechanism behind the relationship between type 1 diabetes and Down's syndrome is still unknown. Management of type 1 diabetes in individuals with Down's syndrome may require less insulin because of more regular, less complex lifestyles compared to the general population.[2] However, glycemic control can still be difficult to achieve in individuals with Down's syndrome because of increased reliance on caregivers and unclear glycemic targets. Furthermore, in our patient, an inability to express symptoms of hypoglycemia put him at high risk of complications, such as loss of consciousness and seizures.

In individuals with type 1 diabetes on MDI insulin, CGM had proven efficacy in improving glycemic control, as measured by HbA_{1c} and TIR, along with reduction of hypoglycemia.[3,4] Recently, an expert panel developed clinical recommendations for glycemic targets based on 14-day CGM data highlighting the importance of TIR and hypoglycemia in guiding management.[5] Different target goals are defined based on type of diabetes, health status, and pregnancy.

Table 30.1—Use of CGM improved patient's glycemic control as seen by lower HbA_{1c}, increased TIR, and decreased TBR

	Initial RT-CGM	Follow-up RT-CGM
HbA_{1c} (%)	8.1	7.5
Average glucose (mg/dL)	165	169
TBR <70 mg/dL (%)	7	1
TIR 70–180 mg/dL (%)	49	58
Time above range >180 mg/dL (%)	44	41
CV (%)	40	32

In "high-risk" populations, where risk of hypoglycemia and its complications is higher, targets allow for less stringent glucose control through reducing the TIR goal to >50% and TBR goal to <1%. Notably, individuals with type 1 diabetes and intellectual disability, such as Down's syndrome, are not discussed, but we could argue that target goals may be similar to those of a high-risk population.

Our patient initially had fair glycemic control, as measured by HbA_{1c} of 8.1%, but he also had frequent hypoglycemia. This result highlights the limitation of relying solely on HbA_{1c} to assess glucose control, because it does not capture time in hypoglycemia or glucose excursions. Initial CGM readings confirmed presence of both high glucose variability and hypoglycemia, likely due to variable food intake and physical activity mismatched with insulin doses. Starting the patient on CGM empowered his caregivers to monitor glucose levels more closely and make appropriate diabetes management decisions throughout the day, reducing both glucose variability and hypoglycemia.

Our case underscores the feasibility and utility of CGM to improve glycemic control and reduce time in hypoglycemia in individuals with type 1 diabetes and intellectual disability, such as Down's syndrome, thus reducing the risk of acute and long-term complications of diabetes. Furthermore, CGM empowers the caregivers of individuals with type 1 diabetes and intellectual disability to manage glucose levels. However, there is still limited information on how to best educate caregivers about CGM and what the CGM target goals for this group should be. More research is needed around the appropriate glycemic targets for individuals with type 1 diabetes and intellectual disability, and the best way to use diabetes technologies in this population.

COMMENTARY

The association of Down's syndrome with diabetes is not uncommon, but, nevertheless, each case presents therapeutic challenges. This case highlights two main points. First is the importance of excellent diabetes education for caregivers, both among family members and at the patient's day care facility. This point proved to be the key for successful implementation of the second major point—initiation and continuation of CGM. As is evident from Table 30.1, CGM allowed the patient to improve his TIR, minimize the time in hypoglycemia, and limit the time above range and glycemic variability with improved HbA_{1c}, even though the average blood glucose levels remained the same. The case clearly demonstrates feasibility of using CGM in people with intellectual disability who have good support in their caregiving environment.

Boris Draznin, MD, PhD

REFERENCES

1. Bergholdt R, Eising S, Nerup J, Pociot F. Increased prevalence of Down's syndrome in individuals with type 1 diabetes in Denmark: a nationwide population-based study. *Diabetologia* 2006;49:1179–1182

2. Rohrer TR, Hennes P, Thon A, et al. Down's syndrome in diabetic patients aged <20 years: an analysis of metabolic status, glycaemic control and autoimmunity in comparison with type 1 diabetes. *Diabetologia* 2010;53:1070–1075

3. Beck RW, Riddlesworth T, Ruedy K, et al. Effect of continuous glucose monitoring on glycemic control in adults with type 1 diabetes using insulin injections: the DIAMOND Randomized Clinical Trial. *JAMA* 2017;317:371–378

4. Lind M, Polonsky W, Hirsch IB, et al. Continuous glucose monitoring vs conventional therapy for glycemic control in adults with type 1 diabetes treated with multiple daily insulin injections: the GOLD Randomized Clinical Trial. *JAMA* 2017;317:379–387

5. Battelino T, Danne T, Bergenstal RM, et al. Clinical targets for continuous glucose monitoring data interpretation: recommendations from the International Consensus on Time in Range. *Diabetes Care* 2019;42:1593–1603

Case 31

A Novel Approach to Achieve Target Time in Range When Using U-500 Regular Insulin in a Continuous Subcutaneous Insulin Infusion (CSII) Pump

Patricia A. Montesinos, NP, CDE,[1] and Michelle F. Magee, MD, MBBCh, BAO, LRCPSI[1,2]

A 58-year-old African American male had type 2 diabetes and insulin resistance with persistent dysglycemia characterized by high glucose variability and suboptimal blood glucose time in range (TIR) (42.5%). His past medical history was remarkable for hypertension, hyperlipidemia, stage 3–4 chronic kidney disease, peripheral neuropathy, gastroparesis, and coronary artery and peripheral vascular disease.

His type 2 diabetes was managed using U-500 regular (U-500R) insulin via continuous subcutaneous insulin infusion (CSII). He monitored blood glucose using a continuous glucose monitoring (CGM) system. His HbA_{1c} ranged from 9.7 to 10.2% over the past year. Other antihyperglycemic agent options were limited or contraindicated by his comorbidities. During past visits, he was noted to have postprandial hyperglycemia (particularly after dinner) as well as late-nocturnal and fasting hypoglycemia. To address the post-dinner hyperglycemia, he had restricted carbohydrates to 60 g, progressively reduced his insulin-to-carbohydrate ratio, reduced the fat in his diet, and activated his meal pre-bolus 30 min before eating. The overnight basal rate had also been reduced to attenuate nocturnal hypoglycemia, and active insulin time was increased from 4 to 6 h to reduce insulin stacking. Despite these adjustments, high glucose variability persisted, and he was unable to achieve a TIR target of >70%.

He weighed 278 lb. His total daily dose of insulin (Tddi) averaged 195 units/day, or 1.55 units/kg/day. Current insulin pump settings (mathematically converted for use of U-500 in a U-100 CSII pump) are as follows: blood glucose target = 140 mg/dL; basal rates = 12:00 A.M. to 3:00 A.M. 0.6 units/h, 3:00 A.M. to 8:00 A.M. 0.8 units/h, 8:00 A.M. to 12:00 A.M. 1.1 units/h; insulin-to-carbohydrate ratio = 1:9 delivered 30 min before meals; insulin sensitivity factor = 1:50; and active insulin time = 6 h. His current CGM data reports are shown in Figures 31.1 and 31.2.

There are reports in the literature that support use of U-500R insulin for CSII therapy.[1–3] The Evaluating U-500R Infusion Versus Injection in Type 2

---

[1]MedStar Diabetes Institute. [2]Georgetown University School of Medicine, Washington, DC

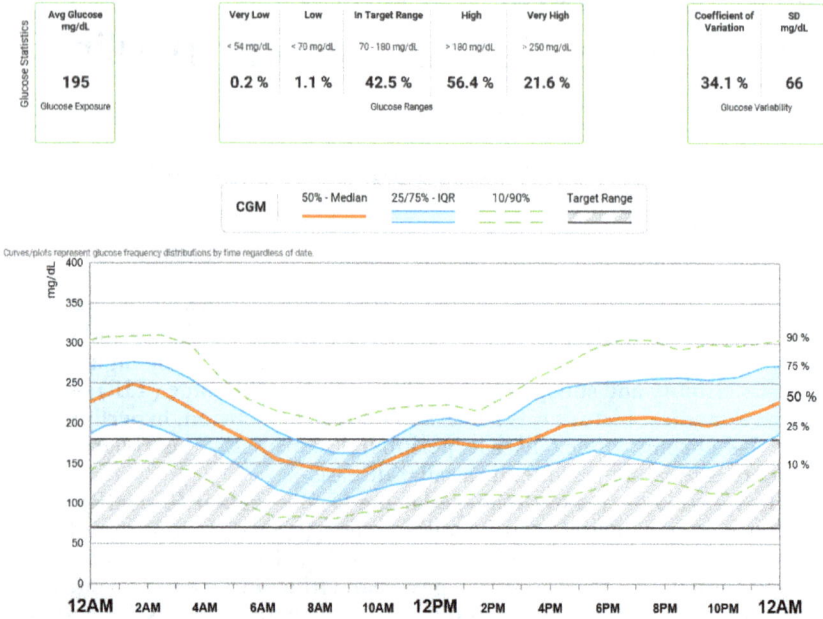

Figure 31.1—Ambulatory glucose profile pre-intervention on U-500R insulin alone via CSII pump.

Diabetes (VIVID) study, which was recently published, is the first randomized controlled trial comparing U-500R by CSII pump to U-500R insulin administered by multiple daily injection (MDI) in patients requiring high-dose insulin (total daily dose >200 to ≤600 units). This study provides guidance for determining CSII settings when U-500R insulin is used. The protocol specified how TDDi U-500R insulin should be distributed and offered three bolus options. TDDi was divided into a 50:50 bolus: basal distribution. In turn, the basal insulin was split into two rates: 6:00 A.M. to 9:00 P.M. at the calculated basal rate and 9:00 P.M. to 6:00 A.M. with a 10% reduction. Up to four basal rates were

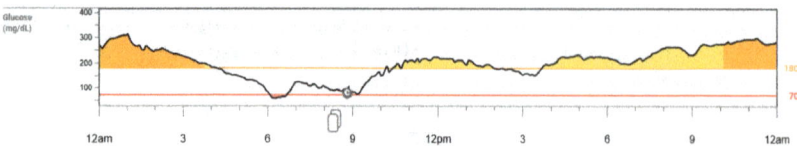

Figure 31.2—An example of a daily report during this time period.

allowed. A bedtime snack without an insulin bolus to prevent nocturnal hypoglycemia was encouraged. The bolus calculator was used to determine meal boluses using one of three options: fixed bolus (40:30:30 for breakfast, lunch, and dinner), carbohydrate (CHO) counting, or meal size per participant estimate, with small = 30 g carbohydrate, medium = 60 g carbohydrate, and large = 90 g carbohydrate. For the latter options, the suggested starting insulin-to-carbohydrate ratio was programmed between 1:3 and 1:5 units/g, with customization allowed. Duration of insulin onboard was 6 h. The reported mean changes from baseline HbA_{1c} were −1.27% in the CSII group and −0.87% with MDI ($P < 0.001$), and 28.7% of the CSII group compared to 18.4% of the MDI group achieved an HbA_{1c} target of <7% ($P < 0.015$). Weight changes and symptomatic and severe hypoglycemia were similar between groups; however, the CSII group had a higher rate of nocturnal hypoglycemia, despite the bedtime snack recommendation.[1]

Glycemic management in this patient affords the opportunity to consider the use of U-500R insulin in CSII therapy, potential limitations to that approach, and a practical solution that has enabled marked improvement in glycemic control in this patient. The time to onset of action of subcutaneously administered U-500R insulin ranges from 30 to 45 min to up to 2.5 h. Its reported mean duration of action is 21 h (range 13–24 h).[3] The CGM data suggest that the U-500R posed a challenge when used as a premeal bolus for this patient, since numerous adjustments in his insulin and dietary regimen to optimize his postmeal glucose levels led to recurrent nocturnal hypoglycemia. This observation was consistent with the reported higher rate of nocturnal hypoglycemia seen in the VIVID study.[1]

Despite intensive efforts to optimize the CSII regimen, sole use of U-500R insulin via the pump did not enable achievement of targeted glycemic control. An alternative solution was needed.

Addition of subcutaneous faster-acting insulin aspart (FiAsp), with a quicker time to onset and shorter duration of action, was explored to address both the 1- to 4-h postprandial hyperglycemia and the 5- to 12-h late-nocturnal and fasting hypoglycemia patterns associated with U-500R insulin CSII use alone.

FiAsp has an onset of action that is twice as fast as that of insulin aspart and mimics physiologic insulin better than rapid-acting insulins.[4] Relevant to this case, the ONSET 2 trial determined that FiAsp provided improved 1-h postprandial glucose with overall rates of hypoglycemia similar to insulin aspart, except for slightly increased risk of 0- to 2-h postprandial hypoglycemia for FiAsp in type 2 diabetes.[5]

The patient started FiAsp by subcutaneous shot for his meal boluses using an insulin-to-carbohydrate ratio of 1:2, mathematically converted from U-500 to U-100 insulin.

The U-500R in the CSII pump now serves solely as basal insulin. This occurrence obviates the need for a meal bolus via the CSII pump well ahead of a meal, which is inconvenient to accommodate and, in this case, was not long enough to allow for time to onset of the bolus of U-500R to attenuate his

Glucose Statistics	Avg Glucose mg/dL		Very Low < 54 mg/dL	Low < 70 mg/dL	In Target Range 70 - 180 mg/dL	High > 180 mg/dL	Very High > 250 mg/dL		Coefficient of Variation	SD mg/dL
	161		**0.0 %**	**0.7 %**	**71.3 %**	**27.9 %**	**6.8 %**		**31.1 %**	**50**
	Glucose Exposure				Glucose Ranges				Glucose Variability	

CGM — 50% - Median 25/75% - IQR 10/90% Target Range

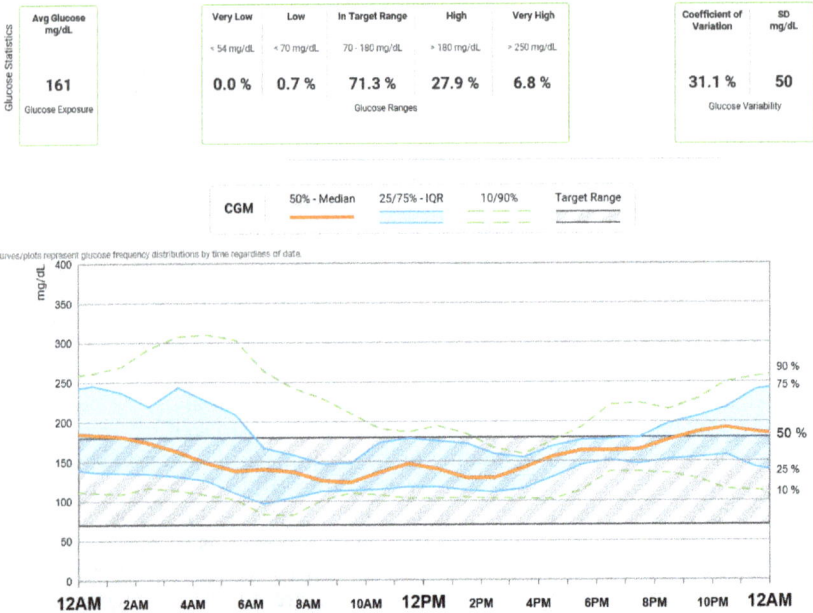

Curves/plots represent glucose frequency distributions by time regardless of date.

Figure 31.3—Ambulatory glucose profile post-intervention on U-500R via CSII pump plus FiAsp before meals.

postmeal hyperglycemia. The patient's CGM reports on the new dual-insulin regimen are shown in Figures 31.3 and 31.4.

With its quicker onset and shorter duration of action, subcutaneous FiAsp for premeal boluses has achieved postprandial glucose targets without increasing risk for hypoglycemia 5–12 h post-bolus. The dual insulins and dual modality of delivery regimen have facilitated a marked improvement in average glucose (195 mg/dL premeal to 161 mg/dL postmeal), SD (66 to 50), and achievement of 72% TIR with minimal hypoglycemia risk and/or blood glucose levels under <70 mg/dL. This TIR would be expected to allow attainment of an HbA_{1c} of 7%. In comparison, the sole use of U-500R insulin for CSII

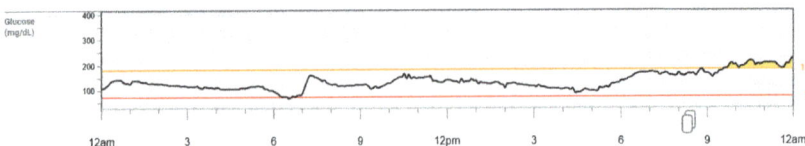

Figure 31.4—An example of a daily report during this time period.

in the VIVID study enabled only a modest percentage (28.7%) of subjects to attain an HbA$_{1c}$ of 7%.

This anecdotal case report suggests that an alternative strategy using subcutaneous ultra-rapid-acting insulin to match meal insulin requirements may be considered to enable targeted glycemic control in patients with type 2 diabetes and insulin resistance who are treated with U-500R insulin via CSII pump.

COMMENTARY

This case demonstrates a successful conversion of U-500 insulin administration to U-100 in an obese insulin-resistant individual using improved dietary compliance and FiAsp. Even though it is not quite clear why this person was on U-500 insulin to begin with, interventions offered by the authors were very successful. One point requires a bit of caution—if this man had significant gastroparesis, a faster-acting premeal insulin could lead to hypoglycemia.

Anne Peters, MD

REFERENCES

1. Grunberger G, Bhargava A, Ly T, et al. Human regular U-500 insulin via continuous subcutaneous insulin infusion versus multiple daily injections in adults with type 2 diabetes: the VIVID study. *Diabetes Obes Metab* 2020;22:434–441. doi: 10.1111/dom.13947

2. McCall AL. U-500 insulin pump case. In *Diabetes Case Studies: Real Problems, Practical Solutions.* Draznin B, Ed. Alexandria, VA, American Diabetes Association, 2015, p. 105–108. doi 10.2337/9781580405713

3. Reutrakul S, Wroblewski K, Brown RL. Clinical use of U-500 regular insulin: review and meta-analysis. *J Diabetes Sci Technol* 2012;6:412–420. doi:10.1177/193229681200600229

4. Davis A, Kuriakose J, Clements J. Faster insulin aspart: a new bolus option for diabetes mellitus. *Clin Pharmacokinet* 2018:58:421–430

5. Bowering K, Case C, Harvey J, et al. Faster aspart versus insulin aspart as part of a basal-bolus regimen in inadequately controlled type 2 diabetes: the ONSET 2 trial. *Diabetes Care* 2017;40:951–957

Automated Insulin Infusion System Is Useful to Control Blood Glucose Concentration During Major Stress in Patients With Type 1 Diabetes

Renzo Cordera, MD,[1] and Davide Maggi, MD, PhD[1]

The patient is a 54-year-old female with longstanding (37 years) type 1 diabetes complicated by acropathy and nonproliferative retinopathy. For years, her blood glucose control has been suboptimal, with HbA_{1c} ranging from 7.8–8.6% along with hypoglycemia. Seven months prior, she began using the MiniMed 670G to infuse insulin with improved glucose control, as reflected by time in range and HbA_{1c}.

Working as a hospital-based radiologist, she contracted the SARS-CoV-2 virus. Her clinical course was characterized by high fever >103.1°F for several days, vomiting, extreme fatigue, and dyspnea. She continued using the MiniMed 670G to control her glycemia: this automated system does not require pump setting change, and it automatically calculates basal insulin doses by predicting glucose concentrations. The patient did not need to set any new parameters and was only required to input the amount of carbohydrates she was eating. The patient was quarantined at home, and her eating was erratic, but she did not require intravenous fluids.

Clinical case reports usually deal with a challenging diagnosis. In this case, the diagnosis was clear: a patient with T1D who contracted SARS-CoV-2 infection. Herein, we describe the clinical performance of a hybrid closed-loop insulin pump that incorporates an automated glucose-sensing device with the pump to infuse insulin in physiologically stressful conditions in a patient with Type 1 diabetes.

Automated insulin delivery systems were developed to circumvent or at least to minimize problems with insulin delivery and algorithms for insulin injections and to be able to integrate glucose concentration, speed of glucose changes, anticipated future glucose values, and other variables.

Today's automated insulin delivery system predicts blood glucose levels and calculates the amount of insulin to be delivered by the pump—a substantial change in insulin therapy. MiniMed 670G (Medtronic) is one of the most sophisticated commercially available insulin infusion systems that control blood glucose independent of the patient's intervention but requires accurate carbohydrate counting and possibly correction doses of insulin for prolonged hyperglycemia.[2] This system is based on algorithms that predict blood glucose

[1]Department of Internal Medicine, University of Genova and Policlinico San Martino, Genova, Italy.

 DOI: 10.2337/9781580407663.32

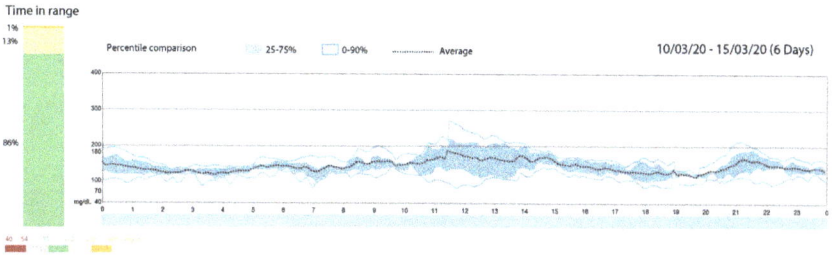

Figure 32.1—Glycemic trend and time in range observed in the 5 days of high fever (>103.1°F) and constitutional symptoms. Data are presented as the mean hourly glucose concentration and time in range (shaded area). It is evident that even under these challenging conditions, the MiniMed 670G maintained excellent and stable glucose control in this patient. It is worth noting that glucose was stable even in the presence of several causes for an inflammatory response, responsible for insulin resistance during infections.

concentration and stabilize glycemia in a safe and desired range. This technology is changing the strategy of insulin therapy from corrective (insulin is injected after glucose increases) protocols to preventive (insulin is infused before glucose increases) protocols. This system (as well as any continuous glucose monitoring) offers the opportunity to evaluate glycemic time in range as a marker of good control, instead of and beyond HbA_{1c}. Thus far, experience with MiniMed 670G has been mainly reported in patients with type 1 diabetes in stable condition. Less is known about the performance of MiniMed 670G during illnesses, such as in the presence of serious intercurrent infections or trauma.

This case illustrates the performance of the MiniMed 670G integrated system in a patient with type 1 diabetes and coronavirus disease 2019 (COVID-19) infection. Although this particular patient was not hospitalized and was treated at home, the stress of a severe acute infection activates systemic inflammation, leading to insulin resistance, unpredictable eating pattern, fever, nausea, and vomiting, among other factors resulting in blood glucose instability, with a significant risk of hypoglycemia presenting a difficult challenge for patients.[1] Hyperglycemia (with or without diabetes) may in and of itself negatively contribute to grave prognosis. A stable blood glucose concentration below 10 mmol/L (180 mg/dL) is the recommended target and a clinical priority in hospitalized patients. In this setting, insulin therapy is mandatory but may not be easy to implement and frequently requires an expert clinical team.[2] Alternatively, a smart automated system for insulin delivery can be used.

In this case, we describe a patient with type 1 diabetes and COVID-19 infection in whom successful glucose control was obtained with the help of a MiniMed 670G, a hybrid closed-loop device. Automatic insulin delivery is a revolutionary advance in insulin therapy, and we describe use of the MiniMed 670G to control blood glucose concentrations in the setting of acute medical stress.

We suggest that automated glucose control and insulin delivery devices should be offered to all patients with type 1 diabetes as the best available mode of therapy, not only for improvement in time in range, but also to improve glycemic responses to stress. This latter point might dramatically change quality of life of people with type 1 diabetes during intercurrent illness.

COMMENTARY

Undoubtedly, diabetes technology has improved our ability to control glycemia while minimizing the risk of hypoglycemia in many patients with type 1 diabetes and patients with type 2 diabetes using insulin. Hybrid closed-loop system devices march in the front row of these great technological advances. While not without problems and shortcomings, these devices have moved the entire field of diabetes management miles ahead.

This particular case describes benefits of the hybrid closed-loop system in a patient with type 1 diabetes and COVID-19. Luckily for this patient, she was not gravely ill and continued to manage her diabetes with a MiniMed 670G insulin pump in the ambulatory setting. This case proves the great utility of this system in a patient under significant stress as a result of severe intercurrent illness. "All's well that ends well" in this case, but hopefully, the use of hybrid closed-loop systems will expand while the science and technology move even farther into the world of common use of the artificial pancreas.

Anne Peters, MD, and Boris Draznin, MD, PhD

REFERENCES

1. American Diabetes Association. 7. Diabetes technology: *Standards of Medical Care in Diabetes—2021. Diabetes Care* 2021;44(Suppl. 1):S85–S99. doi: 10.2337/ dc21-S007

2. Bassetti M, Vena A, Giacobbe DR. The novel Chinese coronavirus (2019-nCoV) infections: challenges for fighting the storm. *Eur J Clin Invest* 2020;50:e13209. doi: 10.1111/eci. 13209

3. Aleppo G, Webb KM. Integrated insulin pumps and continuous glucose monitoring technology in diabetes care today: a perspective of real-life experience with the MiniMed 670G hybrid closed-loop system. *Endocr Pract* 2018;24: 684–692

4. Gupta R, Ghosh A, Singh AK, Misra A. Clinical consideration for patients with diabetes in times of COVID-19 epidemics. *Diabetes Metab Syndr* 2020;14: 211–212

Case 33

Detecting Patterns in Continuous Glucose Monitoring of Glucocorticoid-Treated Patients With Diabetes

Harjyot Sandhu, MD,[1] Janice L. Gilden, MS, MD,[1,2] and Lynne Wentz, MHS, BSN, CDCES[1]

A 76-year-old male with type 2 diabetes complicated by retinopathy and hypertension, with hypothyroidism and interstitial pulmonary fibrosis (requiring home oxygen therapy), underwent continuous glucose monitoring (CGM) for 2 weeks to optimize blood glucose control. The most recent HbA_{1c} was 7.6%. The therapeutic regimen included insulin (30 units detemir in the morning and 50 units detemir in the evening, and mealtime aspart of 22 units with breakfast, 18 units with lunch, and 25 units with dinner, as well as 500 mg metformin p.o. twice daily). During the 2-week period, he was noted to have multiple episodes of mainly asymptomatic preprandial hypoglycemia (Figure 33.1). The average blood glucose levels for the first 10 days on CGM ranged from 123 to 154 mg/dL, with blood glucose levels below 80 mg/dL about 5–28% of the time (Figure 33.1A). He then developed an acute flare-up of interstitial pulmonary fibrosis in the second half of the study period, and 10 mg prednisone p.o. daily was required on the last 2 days of monitoring, which resulted in hyperglycemia. After starting oral prednisone therapy, postprandial blood glucose elevations were noted, and average blood glucose values ranged from 85 to 238 mg/dL, with no hypoglycemic episodes (Figure 33.1B).

The seminal publication in 1949 by Hench et al. reporting that glucocorticoids produced a clinical benefit in patients with rheumatoid arthritis changed the outlook for patients with an inflammatory illness.[1] One year later, Hench was awarded the Nobel Prize in Physiology or Medicine along with Edward Jenner and Thaddeus Reichstein, who first identified the endogenous glucocorticoid cortisol. Glucocorticoids are now recognized to be potent anti-inflammatory agents that modulate many components of the inflammatory cascade via genomic and non-genomic mechanisms. Despite the development of a range of other pharmaceutical and biologic agents that reduce inflammation, glucocorticoids remain a critical part of the therapeutic armamentarium for a wide range of inflammatory and autoimmune diseases, and, currently, glucocorticoid use is increasing.

[1]Diabetes/Endocrinology Section, Chicago Medical School at Rosalind Franklin University of Medicine and Science. [2]Captain James A. Lovell Federal Health Care Center, North Chicago, Illinois.

DOI: 10.2337/9781580407663.33

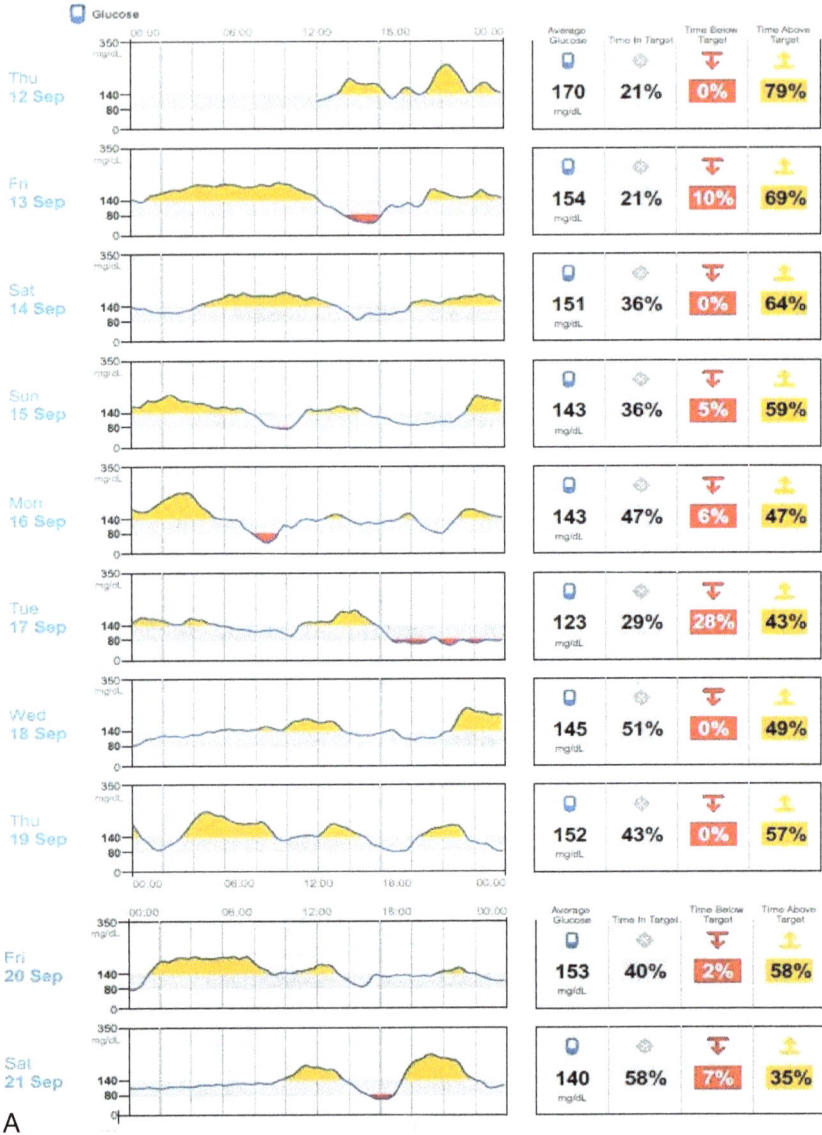

Figure 33.1—CGM report before (*A*) and after (*B*) prednisone use.

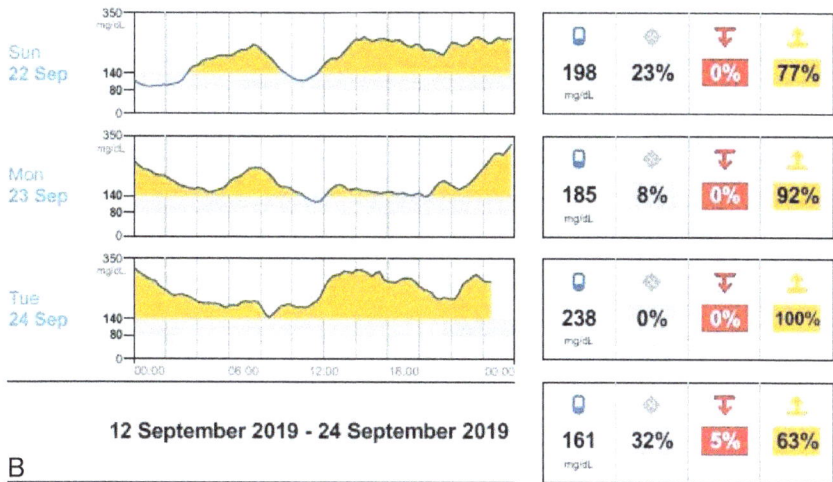

Sun
22 Sep

🔋	✦	🔻	👤
198 mg/dL	23%	0%	77%

Mon
23 Sep

🔋	✦	🔻	👤
185 mg/dL	8%	0%	92%

Tue
24 Sep

🔋	✦	🔻	👤
238 mg/dL	0%	0%	100%

12 September 2019 - 24 September 2019

🔋	✦	🔻	👤
161 mg/dL	32%	5%	63%

B

Figure 33.1 — *(continued)*

Early studies have reported that glucocorticoid therapy can increase blood glucose concentrations. However, almost 70 years after their first use, the indications for treatment of glucocorticoid-induced hyperglycemia and optimum therapeutic approach remain unclear. Management of this large group of patients depends on extrapolated data from other clinical scenarios, combined with an understanding of the pharmacokinetics and pharmacodynamics of glucocorticoids and of antihyperglycemic agents.

Glucocorticoids are most commonly prescribed as the semi-synthetic formulation prednisone, which is usually administered as a single morning dose. Prednisone therapy is usually prescribed in two main patterns. It can be prescribed short term in medium-high doses to treat an acute inflammatory illness, such as an exacerbation of interstitial pulmonary fibrosis. Prednisone is also prescribed long term at lower doses, usually <10 mg/day, to attenuate chronic inflammatory disease progression. Similar glucocorticoid doses are also prescribed to prevent rejection after solid organ transplant and in patients needing glucocorticoid replacement therapy.

Glucocorticoid-induced hyperglycemia is the result of impairment of multiple pathways affecting carbohydrate metabolism (Table 33.1).[2] Glucocorticoids induce peripheral insulin resistance, which predominantly reflects insulin action in skeletal muscle.[3] At higher doses, glucocorticoids impair oxidative and non-oxidative glucose disposal, whereas in patients on long-term low-dose prednisone, non-oxidative glucose disposal is predominantly reduced. Glucocorticoids reduce glycogen synthase activity in skeletal muscle, which contributes to a reduction in peripheral non-oxidative glucose disposal. Other aspects of carbohydrate metabolism are also affected. Glucocorticoids cause hepatic

Table 33.1—Mechanisms of glucocorticoid-induced diabetes

Reduced peripheral insulin sensitivity and/or promotion of weight gain
Increase in glucose production through promotion of hepatic gluconeogenesis
Destruction of pancreatic cells, leading to β-cell injury (inflammation)
β-Cell dysfunction
Impaired insulin release
Inhibited glyceroneogenesis
Increase in fatty acids

insulin resistance, resulting in increased hepatic glucose output, even during long-term, low-dose prednisone therapy. Acutely, glucocorticoids also reduce insulin secretion, but insulin secretion is not reduced in patients on long-term, low-dose prednisone. An acute reduction in incretin-induced insulin secretion is likely to contribute to the observed reduction in insulin secretion with glucocorticoids.

CGM systems are increasingly used to optimize management of diabetes in the outpatient setting. CGM measures interstitial glucose concentrations, which closely approximates plasma glucose after a short time lag, every 5 min for up to 14 days. CGM provides detailed information regarding nocturnal and postprandial glycemia, whereas standard fingerstick blood glucose monitoring regimens do not. As such, CGM has the potential to provide great insight into the glycemic effect of glucocorticoid therapy.

Endogenous glucocorticoid excess in Cushing's syndrome predominantly increases postprandial blood glucose concentration, with fasting blood glucose often in the normal range. If exogenous glucocorticoids cause a similar pattern of hyperglycemia, current conventional strategies may inadequately treat postprandial hyperglycemia, and use of long-acting basal insulin may precipitate nocturnal hypoglycemia. Avoidance of severe hypoglycemia is important because it has been implicated as a potential cause of increased mortality in patients receiving intensive insulin therapy. However, few studies have provided a detailed analysis of the effect of various glucocorticoids with different half-lives on blood glucose concentration to optimize treatment of glucocorticoid-induced hyperglycemia.

There are studies that have used CGM to provide a detailed analysis of the frequency and pattern of hyperglycemia induced by prednisone in patients hospitalized with an exacerbation of chronic obstructive pulmonary disorder (COPD).[4] The studies have demonstrated that glucose concentrations during CGM in glucocorticoid-treated subjects and a well-matched control group diverge at midday, with blood glucose levels ~20% higher after lunch and dinner. When prednisolone was administered in the morning, the peak glucose occurred about 8 h after prednisone administration, a similar time frame to that in which the maximal inhibition of lymphocyte proliferation develops. If prednisolone was taken later in the day, the mean glucose peak occurred after 5 h, so the time period of glucose elevation was similar to that after morning administration. The effect of prednisolone then wears off overnight, with an almost identical mean glucose concentration between midnight and noon.

Our findings have important implications for clinical practice. First, glucocorticoid-treated patients should be educated regarding the importance of checking capillary blood glucose concentration (or wearing a CGM device) after lunch and before and after dinner, because reliance on measurement of morning blood glucose is likely to underestimate prednisone-induced hyperglycemia. Second, glucose-lowering therapy should be predominantly directed at the time period between midday and midnight. Caution should be exercised with the use of long-acting basal insulin, because it may precipitate nocturnal hypoglycemia when the effect of prednisone wanes. Because the first glucose excursion begins on average 3 h after prednisone administration, higher insulin doses at lunch and dinner are likely to be required. Furthermore, CGM can be used to evaluate the effects of varying glucocorticoids on glycemic control in patients with diabetes.

Because of differences in steroid dose and the scheme used, the approach to hyperglycemia should always be individualized.[5] A complete evaluation of the degree of preexisting glucose intolerance; the patient's clinical condition; the degree of hyperglycemia; the type, dose, and frequency of administration of the corticosteroid compound; and the mechanism of action, pharmacokinetics, and pharmacodynamics of the different antihyperglycemic agents must be made to determine the best treatment approach in each patient. In our opinion, when selecting the best treatment, the first consideration to make is whether to prescribe oral/injectable antihyperglycemic drugs or insulin (Figure 33.2).[5]

COMMENTARY

Use of steroids in patients with diabetes for a variety of medical reasons is widespread. While the use of NPH insulin instead of a longer-acting basal insulin to counteract glucocorticoid-induced hyperglycemia is well accepted by most diabetologists, I think the first step is to determine whether the hyperglycemia associated with steroid use requires additional treatment at all, or is it just a transient issue. Additionally, adjusting preexisting insulin doses, as in this case, is different from starting insulin or other agents. The common practice is to taper insulin (especially if NPH was added to previous insulin regimen) as the steroid doses are tapered to avoid hypoglycemia. Finally, the case illustrates that CGM can be extremely important in helping with management of patients with steroid-induced hyperglycemia.

Anne Peters, MD

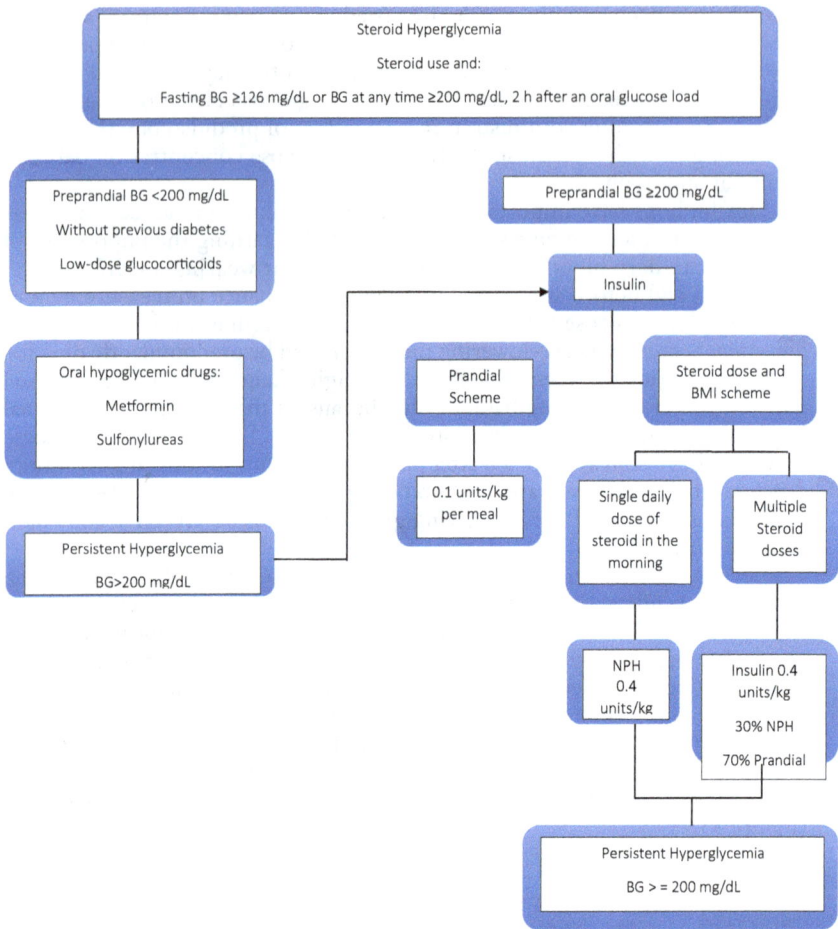

Figure 33.2—Adapted from Tamez-Pérez et al.[5] Algorithm for the management of glucocorticoid-induced hyperglycemia is shown. Glargine and other analogs can be recommended in cases of nocturnal hyperglycemia associated with long-acting steroid use. BG, blood glucose.

REFERENCES

1. Radhakutty A, Burt M. Management of endocrine disease: critical review of the evidence underlying management of glucocorticoid-induced hyperglycaemia. *Eur J Endocrinol* 2018;179:R207–R218

2. Suh S, Park MK. Glucocorticoid-induced diabetes mellitus: an important but overlooked problem. *Endocrinol Metab (Seoul)* 2017;32:180–189. doi:10.3803/EnM.2017.32.2.180

3. Rizza RA, Mandarino LF, Gerich JE. Cortisol-induced insulin resistance in man: impaired suppression of glucose production and stimulation of glucose utilization due to a postreceptor defect of insulin action. *J Clin Endocrinol Metab* 1982;54:131–138

4. Burt MG, Roberts GW, Aguilar-Loza NR, Frith P, Stranks SN. Continuous monitoring of circadian glycemic patterns in patients receiving prednisolone for COPD. *J Clin Endocrinol Metab* 2011;96;1789–1796

5. Tamez-Pérez HE, Quintanilla-Flores DL, Rodríguez-Gutiérrez R, González-González JG, Tamez-Peña AL. Steroid hyperglycemia: Prevalence, early detection and therapeutic recommendations: a narrative review. *World J Diabetes* 2015;6:1073–1081. doi:10.4239/wjd.v6.i8.1073

Part 6

Hypoglycemia

Case 34

Hyperinsulemic Hypoglycemia After Roux-en-Y Gastric Bypass Surgery: Both Fasting and Postprandial

Maria Magar, MD,[1] Anne Peters, MD,[2] and Braden Barnett, MD[3]

The case subject is a 34-year-old female with a past history of Roux-en-Y gastric bypass (RYGB) surgery for obesity (BMI 41 kg/m^2). Two years after the RYGB, now with BMI of 24.9 kg/m^2, she started having symptomatic hypoglycemia, nausea, and vomiting. An inpatient 72-h fast was negative, but she experienced a drop in her blood glucose (BG) from 20 to 50 mg/dL, with concurrent loss of consciousness after eating a mixed meal. She was subsequently diagnosed with post–gastric bypass hypoglycemia and was discharged on acarbose and a high-protein, low-carbohydrate diet. One month later, she had a laparoscopic-assisted gastric bypass revision and was able to drink fruit juice and protein shakes without hypoglycemia at discharge.

One week after discharge, she again experienced postprandial hypoglycemia and started to also develop fasting hypoglycemia. During a repeat 72-h fast, her BG dropped to 47 mg/dL, and a C-peptide at that time was 0.6 ng/mL (normal range 0.8–3.5 ng/mL), proinsulin was 1.7 pmol/L (normal ≤8 pmol/L), and insulin level was 2 µIU/mL (normal range 3–19 µIU/mL). A computed tomography (CT) scan of the abdomen with pancreas protocol, an endoscopic ultrasound, and a selective arterial calcium stimulation test with hepatic vein sampling were negative for insulinoma. The patient was discharged on diazoxide and octreotide, which had improved her hypoglycemia during the hospitalization. Although she took both medications consistently (octreotide to a lesser extent, since it gave her severe nausea) as well as adhering to a protein-enriched diet, she continued to report hypoglycemia at an outpatient follow-up appointment.

Given her refractory symptoms, the patient underwent a partial pancreatectomy ~4 years after her initial bariatric surgery. Based on the resulting pathology, she was diagnosed with nesidioblastosis. For 2 months after her surgery, the patient was symptom-free and then started developing episodes of weakness, tremors, slurred speech, and vision loss that would last up to 4 h. Stroke was ruled out at an outside hospital. Per the patient's reports, the symptoms did not seem to be related to or improve with food

---

[1]LAC+USC Medical Center, Los Angeles, California. [2]Keck School of Medicine of the University of Southern California, Los Angeles, California. [3]Keck School of Medicine of the University of Southern California, Los Angeles, California

DOI: 10.2337/9781580407663.34

intake, since her BG levels ranged from 78 to 180 mg/dL at home during the episodes. There were no instances of objective/subjective hypoglycemia during another 72-h fast (BG 84–93 mg/dL) or after a large carbohydrate meal (BG >200 mg/dL). Her aforementioned symptoms were thus felt to be unrelated to her prior gastric surgeries, and she was discharged with metformin 500 mg twice a day. Almost exactly 5 years after her initial RYGB, the patient presented again after losing consciousness with a BG of 30 mg/dL, although she was consistently eating six small, mixed meals a day. It was then decided that she should undergo a total pancreatectomy, after which she was started on glargine 14 units daily and regular insulin 3 units with meals, with no subsequent hypoglycemic episodes as of this writing.

This complex case reflects the difficulty in managing postprandial hyperinsulinemic hypoglycemia, which has increasingly become a known complication of bariatric surgery at large.[1] In particular, our patient had severe recurrent hypoglycemia develop after her RYGB surgery. There are various etiologies for post-RYGB hypoglycemia including insulinoma, late dumping syndrome, and nesidioblastosis as seen in this case. Insulinoma is classically associated with only fasting hypoglycemia, which, interestingly, our patient had in addition to postprandial hypoglycemia—possibly a consequence of elevated glucagon-like peptide (GLP)-1 levels.[2,3] "Late dumping" often occurs years after bariatric surgery and presents as hypoglycemia 1 h or more after a meal. It is thought to be due to exaggerated responses of GLP-1 and insulin to meals. Nesidioblastosis consists of hypertrophy and hyperfunctioning of pancreatic β-cells that classically leads to postprandial hypoglycemia. Pathologic islet hyperplasia and dysplasia as well as β-cell hypertrophy and budding from ductal epithelium are seen.[1]

Nesidioblastosis was initially thought to be only a congenital disorder, but recently it was discovered to develop in adults as well.[1] Around the middle of the 20th century, this condition was first defined by George Laidlaw as the novel development of islets of Langerhans from pancreatic duct epithelium. Although the diagnosis is confirmed by pathology, it is unclear whether the histologic changes of nesidioblastosis are reactive to obesity before surgery or a consequence of the actual surgical intervention. The particular frequency of non-congenital nesidioblastosis is unknown but thought to make up to 10% of organic hyperinsulinism. Nesidioblastosis can be seen with a serum glucose of <40 mg/dL, insulin level >7 μU/mL, and/or a positive 72-h fasting test; however, a histologic examination solidifies the diagnosis as mentioned above and differentiates it from other clinically similar presentations such as insulinoma.[3] The diagnosis can further be supported by symptom improvement after partial pancreatectomy.

Most hyperinsulinemic hypoglycemia can be managed by a low-carbohydrate diet alone or low-carbohydrate mixed meals. If dietary modifications fail, pharmacological agents can especially help mild or moderate cases: α-glucosidase inhibitors, diazoxide, octreotide, or calcium-channel blockers. If these agents do not resolve the hypoglycemia, RYGB reversal or conversion to a sleeve gastrectomy can be done, and it is advised that a period of strict carbohydrate restriction be followed after surgery to decrease incretin secretion. Hypoglycemia can still be refractory after these procedures as in our patient, and thus partial, subtotal, or total pancreatic resection may be warranted.[1] Selective arterial calcium stimulation testing can localize as well as guide the degree of surgical intervention. With extensive pancreatic surgery, the patient will be committed to lifelong insulin.[3]

COMMENTARY

This case illustrates not only reasonably common clinical features of postprandial hypoglycemia in RYGB patients, but also a scrupulous diagnostic approach to these patients and their aggressive management. The patient was thoroughly investigated with multiple 72-h fasts and underwent two pancreatic surgeries (partial and total pancreatectomy) to control her intractable hypoglycemia. She has gone from being an obese individual who was a good candidate for gastric bypass to a person with diabetes (post-pancreatectomy) treated with multiple daily insulin injections. It appears that the diagnosis of nesidioblastosis was firmly established by pathology. In this case, total pancreatectomy seems to be a curative procedure, even though subsequent management of her diabetes will not be easy.

Boris Draznin, MD, PhD

REFERENCES

1. Malik S, Mitchell J, Steffen K, et al. Recognition and management of hyperinsulinemic hypoglycemia after bariatric surgery. *Obes Res Clin Pract* 2016;10: 1–14

2. Chen X, Kamel D, Barnett B, et al. An unusual presentation of post gastric bypass hypoglycemia with both postprandial and fasting hypoglycemia. *Endocrinol Diabetes Metab Case Rep* 2018;18–0089

3. Tharakan G, Behary P, Wewer Albrechtsen NJ, et al. Roles of increased glycaemic variability, GLP-1 and glucagon in hypoglycaemia after Roux-en-Y gastric bypass. *Eur J Endocrinol* 2017;177:455–464

Case 35

Refractory Hypoglycemia Due to Massive Unintentional Insulin Overdose

Jennifer D. Merrill, MD,[1] and Jennifer Rowell, MD[1]

A 30-year-old uninsured male was admitted with status epilepticus in the setting of severe hypoglycemia. He was diagnosed with type 1 diabetes at age 21 years, when he presented with diabetic ketoacidosis and positive GAD antibody (0.82 nmol/L, reference range <0.02). He had no known complications of diabetes but had not seen an outpatient physician in over 1 year. There was no evidence of pharmacy fills of his prescribed insulin regimen. His family noted that the patient never checked his blood glucose at home, but that he did use insulin daily. He had had two encounters with emergency services at outside hospitals in the last year because of hypoglycemia.

The patient had been drinking alcohol most of the day before admission. His friends noted that he had repeatedly given himself bolus injections of an unknown insulin without checking his blood glucose, believing the insulin was not working. He was found unconscious 12 h later and the emergency medical service (EMS) was called.

Alcohol use has been implicated in up to 20% of hospital presentations for hypoglycemia.[1] In studies with continuous glucose monitoring, people with type 1 diabetes who consumed moderate amounts of alcohol have twice the risk of hypoglycemia in the next 24 h.[2] Furthermore, alcohol impairs the hormonal counter-regulatory response to hypoglycemia. Alcohol inhibits gluconeogenesis but not glycogenolysis, so depleted hepatic glycogen stores might potentiate hypoglycemia.

On EMS arrival, his glucose was 10 mg/dL. Glucagon and 50 g dextrose were administered. In route to the hospital, he had a seizure and was treated with midazolam. On arrival, he had another, 7-minute seizure and was given lorazepam twice without response. He was then loaded with fosphenytoin.

He was intubated, sedated with propofol, and transferred to the intensive care unit. A 10% dextrose drip was started at 125 mL/h, but blood glucose remained <30 mg/dL. Dextrose was increased to 20% at 150 mL/h. Glucose was monitored every 30 min. Because the insulin and C-peptide

[1]Duke University Division of Endocrinology, Diabetes and Metabolism, Duke University School of Medicine, Durham, North Carolina.

 DOI: 10.2337/9781580407663.35

142	112	9	
3.7	23	0.9	33

16.4 \ 14.9 / 293

Mg++: 1.6
Phos: 1.8
Ca++: 8.6
Lactate: 17.1
Trop: <0.01
Alb: 3.5

CK: 2087
β-Hydroxybutyrate: undetectable
C-peptide: undetectable
Insulin: 39.0 µIU/mL (normal <23)
HbA$_{1c}$: 9.1

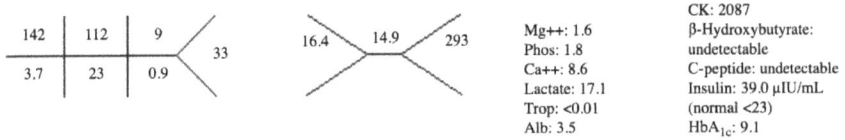

Figure 35.1—Admission labs.

levels were not available until the day after admission, he was started on glucagon and octreotide infusions, as well as stress dose hydrocortisone. He required an additional 100 g dextrose to maintain serum glucose at the >80 mg/dL level (total 550 g dextrose in the first 24 h).

Dextrose is the mainstay of treatment for hypoglycemia. Both intravenous dextrose and oral administration of carbohydrates should be considered.[3] In refractory cases, additional therapies may be considered and can be tailored to the cause of hypoglycemia and capacity for endogenous insulin secretion.

Normally, a decrease in plasma glucose causes a decrease in β-cell insulin secretion that signals an increase in α-cell glucagon secretion during hypoglycemia. In absolute endogenous insulin deficiency, β-cell failure means there is no decrease in β-cell insulin secretion and thus no increase in α-cell glucagon secretion during hypoglycemia. Glucagon increases blood glucose by increasing hepatic glycogenolysis and, with other glucose counter-regulatory hormones, stimulates hepatic gluconeogenesis. A study comparing glycemic profiles after administration of either 1 mg intravenous glucagon or 25 g dextrose in patients with severe hypoglycemia found recovery of normal blood glucose and normal level of consciousness after glucagon was slower than after dextrose.[4] Although administration of glucagon was attempted for our patient, it was unlikely to be effective since the hepatic glycogen stores would have already been depleted.

Octreotide has been used in cases of sulfonylurea overdose to decrease endogenous insulin secretion in response to glucose administration.[3] Octreotide binds to somatostatin-2 receptors located on pancreatic β-cells, which inhibit insulin secretion by preventing calcium influx. Octreotide has been used as a treatment for hypoglycemia due to insulin overdose with the goal of preventing additional insulin release from the pancreas in response to exogenously administered dextrose. This treatment is of little utility in patients with no capacity for endogenous insulin secretion like our patient.

Corticosteroids induce insulin resistance, even at an anti-inflammatory dose, by decreasing peripheral glucose use.[5] The hyperglycemic effect of high-dose corticosteroids can be an adjunctive therapy for refractory hypoglycemia in the setting of massive insulin overdose.

Non-pharmacological therapies have also been attempted for treatment of massive insulin overdose. Although insulin is minimally dialyzable when the gradient is high, hemodialysis is generally considered ineffective because the duration of insulin action depends on the rate of absorption rather than the rate of elimination. Surgical resection of the subcutaneous insulin depot has been successful in case reports,[3] but our patient had no obvious injection sites for consideration of this treatment.

Endocrinology recommended discontinuing octreotide because of the lack of endogenous insulin production. Seizures stopped, but he did not regain consciousness for another 4 days. Glucagon was discontinued on day 2. Stress dose steroids were weaned but not discontinued. Blood glucose was monitored hourly, and dextrose infusion rate was weaned as blood glucose increased to 200 mg/dL and weaned off on day 3. On hospital day 5, insulin level declined to 14.3. On hospital day 4, continuous tube feeds were started and glucose began to trend up. Hyperglycemia was managed with insulin drip. Renal function remained normal throughout the admission. Eventually, the patient regained consciousness but not normal cognitive function. Insulin was transitioned to a basal-bolus regimen as he began to eat.

His fiancée brought a nearly empty, weathered 10-mL vial of U-100 glargine insulin to the hospital. Thus, the insulin he had been using to treat perceived high glucose was actually long-acting basal insulin. He had used this entire vial of insulin the day before admission.

After a massive glargine insulin overdose, our patient with type 1 diabetes continued to have a supraphysiologic insulin level without receiving insulin for 3 days and did not require any additional basal insulin for 4 days. Glargine insulin is modified to be soluble in an acidic environment compared to human insulin. The insulin precipitates in the tissue at a neutral pH in a depot from which it is slowly released. The pharmacokinetics are not known after large overdoses, but case reports all indicate the need for extended glucose infusion to treat the resultant hypoglycemia, which can last up to 120 h and may depend on the insulin dose administered.[3] In our patient, the duration of hypoglycemia was likely exacerbated by the reduced capacity from gluconeogenesis caused by his recent alcohol use.

He was uninsured at discharge, so he was discharged on pre-mixed 70/30 insulin because of cost. Health care coverage was established for him as an outpatient, but he was lost to follow-up.

COMMENTARY

Alcohol abuse and type 1 diabetes is an unfortunate combination, and when it is accompanied by hurdles in access to care because of inadequate health care coverage by private and public insurance, it becomes extremely dangerous, as this case illustrates.

Boris Draznin, MD, PhD

REFERENCES

1. Potter J, Clarke P, Gale EA, Dave SH, Tattersall RB. Insulin-induced hypogly-caemia in an accident and emergency department: the tip of an iceberg? *Br Med J (Clin Res Ed)* 1982;285:1180–1182

2. Richardson T, Weiss M, Thomas P, Kerr D. Day after the night before: influ-ence of evening alcohol on risk of hypoglycemia in patients with type 1 diabetes. *Diabetes Care* 2005;28:1801–1802

3. Johansen NJ, Christensen MB. A systematic review on insulin overdose cases: clinical course, complications and treatment options. *Basic Clin Pharmacol Toxicol* 2018;122:650–659

4. Collier A, Steedman DJ, Patrick AW, et al. Comparison of intravenous glucagon and dextrose in treatment of severe hypoglycemia in an accident and emergency department. *Diabetes Care* 1987;10:712–715

5. Pagano G, Cavallo-Perin P, Cassader M, et al. An in vivo and in vitro study of the mechanism of prednisone-induced insulin resistance in healthy subjects. *J Clin Invest* 1983;72:1814–1820

A Case of Prolonged Hypoglycemia Due to Sulfonylurea and Concurrent Antibiotic Use

Jennifer D. Merrill, MD,[1] and Susan E. Spratt, MD[1]

A 65-year-old African American female with recurrent ER+/PR+/HER2–left breast cancer with metastases to lymph nodes and bone, hypertension, dyslipidemia, and type 2 diabetes presented to the emergency department with refractory hypoglycemia.

She was found unresponsive in the field with a fingerstick glucose of 11 mg/dL. She was given 25 g intravenous dextrose by emergency medical services, with improvement in glucose to ~90 mg/dL. She was brought to the hospital, where vital signs were normal, and exam was unremarkable except for previous left mastectomy and firm matted cervical lymphadenopathy. Admission labs are shown in Figure 36.1.

She developed recurrent hypoglycemia requiring an additional 100 g intravenous dextrose and was started on a D10 infusion at a rate of 150 mL/h and transferred to the medical intensive care unit. C-peptide from admission was 13.5 ng/mL (upper limit of normal 4.5 ng/mL) in the setting of serum glucose of 68 mg/dL. Hours later, concurrent insulin level was 161.2 μ1U/mL (upper limit of normal 23 μIU/mL). Toxicology screen and ethanol level were negative.

She had a >10-year history of diabetes, initially managed with oral medications. She was unable to tolerate metformin due to diarrhea. She had no diabetes complications. Review of her outpatient glucose logs while she was on insulin indicated average glucose of 111 mg/dL (range 45–191 mg/dL) but with hypoglycemia to <70 mg/dL several times per month, usually in the afternoon or early evening. She typically felt adrenergic symptoms of hypoglycemia when her blood glucose level was 55 mg/dL.

Until 4 days before admission, her diabetes had been managed with Humalog pre-mix 75/25 insulin, with 40 units total daily dose 6 months before admission. Insulin was decreased at each outpatient visit due to hypoglycemia, until the most recent visit 4 days before admission when she was transitioned from 10 units of pre-mixed 70/30 insulin to 1 mg glimepiride. She had experienced a 50.7-lb weight loss over the last 4 months, but her weight had recently stabilized at 99.2 lb. She denied any recent use of

---

[1]Duke University Division of Endocrinology, Diabetes and Metabolism, Duke University School of Medicine, Durham, NC

DOI: 10.2337/9781580407663.36

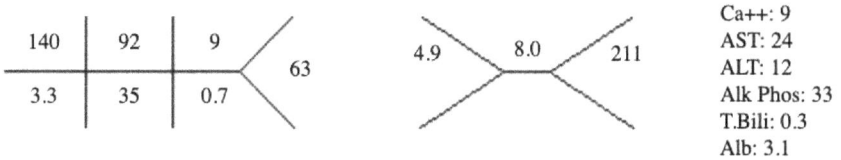

Figure 36.1—Admission labs.

tobacco, illicit substances, or alcohol. She had a family history of type 2 diabetes in her mother, brother, and sister, but no family history of neuro-endocrine tumors.

The day after she saw her outpatient endocrinologist, she saw her primary care doctor for an upper respiratory infection and was prescribed 100 mg doxycycline monohydrate twice daily as well as pseudoephedrine-guaifenesin. Her other medications included abemaciclib, ascorbic acid, aspirin, atorvastatin, benazepril, calcium citrate, doxycycline, ferrous sulfate, glimepiride 1 mg daily with breakfast, and tramadol 50 mg every 6 h as needed. The patient endorsed exact adherence to all of these medications and provided the pill bottle with only three missing tabs of glimepiride, which confirmed that she had taken this exactly as prescribed.

Medication interactions are a commonly overlooked cause of hypoglycemia. A retrospective study of Medicare claims data of patients 66 years or older treated with sulfonylurea for diabetes demonstrated increased risk of hospitalization for hypoglycemia when patients were treated with several commonly prescribed antimicrobials (Table 36.1).[1] Patient factors associated with hypoglycemia included older age, female sex, African American or Hispanic race/ethnicity, higher comorbidity, and antecedent hypoglycemic episode. Antibiotics most associated with hypoglycemia included

Table 36.1—Antimicrobials most often associated with hypoglycemia when combined with sulfonylurea in Medicare patients[1]

Antimicrobial	Odds Ratio (95% CI)
Ciprofloxacin	1.62 (1.33–1.97)
Clarithromycin	3.96 (2.42–6.49)
Fluconazole	0.92 (0.52–1.61)
Levofloxacin	2.60 (2.18–3.10)
Metronidazole	2.11 (1.28–3.47)
Moxifloxacin	1.13 (0.65–1.98)
Trimethoprim-sulfamethoxazole	2.56 (2.12–3.10)

clarithromycin, levofloxacin, trimethoprim-sulfamethoxazole, metronidazole, and ciprofloxacin. In 2009, 28.3% of patients prescribed a sulfonylurea filled a prescription for one of these antimicrobials. Although it was not one of the most commonly associated antimicrobials, doxycycline has been previously reported to cause hypoglycemia in people both with and without diabetes.[2-4] Medications should always be considered in the differential diagnosis for hypoglycemia.[5]

Our patient's recent transition to sulfonylurea from insulin prompted the medical intensive care unit team to start octreotide infusion in addition to the dextrose. Blood glucose was checked every half hour and then at longer intervals as hypoglycemia began to resolve over the next 24 h. Thyroid-stimulating hormone (TSH) was normal and she had a normal 250-μg ACTH stimulation test. Sulfonylurea screen obtained 24 h after the most recent glimepiride dose was negative. Review of a recent computed tomography (CT) scan of the chest, abdomen, and pelvis showed multiple pulmonary nodules measuring up to 3.3 cm, normal thyroid, postsurgical changes of left mastectomy, normal pancreas, and multiple low-attenuation lesions throughout the liver that were too small to characterize. Repeat insulin level was 6.9 μIU/mL and C-peptide was 0.9 ng/mL 36 h later, when serum glucose was 257 mg/dL. Dextrose and octreotide infusions were weaned. The patient was monitored for 24 h off of glucose-lowering medications, and blood glucose remained <200 mg/dL. She was discharged without diabetes medications.

Our patient initially had inappropriately elevated insulin and C-peptide levels, which supported a hypothesis that her hypoglycemia was mediated by endogenous insulin secretion due to sulfonylurea and doxycycline. Additionally, she had multiple liver lesions of the abdomen on her CT scan, which may have contributed to impaired gluconeogenesis. Octreotide was used to bind the G protein–coupled somatostatin receptors on pancreatic β-cells to help inhibit inappropriate insulin secretion.[6] Alternative causes of hypoglycemia were ruled out and insulin and C-peptide had returned to appropriate levels before discharge.

COMMENTARY

The case draws our attention to a seemingly forgotten fact that the combination of sulfonylurea preparations with certain antibiotics can cause hypoglycemia in patients with diabetes. In this particular case, endogenous hyperinsulinemia (elevated C-peptide and insulin) was identified on admission and subsided when the culprit drugs were stopped. Another interesting detail is the use of octreotide to combat increased insulin secretion. This method has been used previously and is probably a good approach to sulfonylurea excess. The take-home message is to always review patients' medications.

Boris Draznin, MD, PhD

REFERENCES

1. Parekh TM, Raji M, Lin YL, Tan A, Kuo YF, Goodwin JS. Hypoglycemia after antimicrobial drug prescription for older patients using sulfonylureas. *JAMA Intern Med* 2014;174:1605–1612

2. Basaria S, Braga M, Moore WT. Doxycycline-induced hypoglycemia in a nondiabetic young man. *South Med J* 2002;95:1353–1354

3. Odeh M, Oliven A. Doxycycline-induced hypoglycemia. *J Clin Pharmacol* 2000;40:1173–1174

4. Kennedy KE, Teng C, Patek TM, Frei CR. Hypoglycemia associated with antibiotics alone and in combination with sulfonylureas and meglitinides: an epidemiologic surveillance study of the FDA Adverse Event Reporting System (FAERS). *Drug Saf* 2020;43:363–369

5. Cryer PE, Axelrod L, Grossman AB, et al. Evaluation and management of adult hypoglycemic disorders: an Endocrine Society Clinical Practice Guideline. *J Clin Endocrinol Metab* 2009;94:709–728

6. Glatstein M, Scolnik D, Bentur Y. Octreotide for the treatment of sulfonylurea poisoning. *Clin Toxicol (Phila)* 2012;50:795–804

Part 7

Cystic Fibrosis–Related Diabetes (CFRD)

Case 37

"Do I Really Need Insulin?" The Role of Insulin Therapy in Cystic Fibrosis– Related Diabetes (CFRD)

Nader Kasim, MD,[1] Antoinette Moran, MD,[2] and Amir Moheet, MD[3]

A 23-year-old female with cystic fibrosis (CF) (homozygous for the F508del mutation), history of pancreatic insufficiency, and history of poor weight gain underwent an oral glucose tolerance test (OGTT) per routine screening for cystic fibrosis–related diabetes (CFRD). She had a fasting glucose of 110 mg/dL (6.1 mmol/L), 1-h OGTT glucose of 191 mg/dL (10.6 mmol/L), and 2-h OGTT glucose of 225 mg/dL (12.5 mmol/L). Her insulin levels were low, as is typical in CF, with a peak insulin level of 45 mU/L during the OGTT. Based on these results, she was diagnosed with CFRD. She was instructed to self-monitor blood glucose values at home. During her follow-up visit, blood glucose logs were reviewed, and she was noted to check approximately 8 times per day. Average blood glucose was 120 mg/dL (6.7 mmol/L), SD 26 mg/dL (1.4 mmol/L). She did not report any symptoms suggestive of hyperglycemia, including polyuria or polydipsia.

The patient experienced ongoing insidious decline in lung function and weight. She was regularly meeting with a dietitian to optimize macronutrient intake and enzyme replacement. In addition, she was working with pulmonology to optimize her lung function. Despite these efforts, pulmonary function and weight declined (Figure 37.1).

Four months after her diagnosis of CFRD, she was started on insulin glargine U-100 5 units daily (indicated by an arrow in Figure 37.1), and the dose was titrated up to 15 units daily (0.25 units/kg) over the following 3 months.

> Although her home blood glucose levels were only modestly elevated, insulin replacement therapy is recommended in CFRD to induce anabolism to improve pulmonary function and weight gain.

Shortly after initiation of insulin therapy, she saw steady improvement in forced expiratory volume (FEV1) and weight. Home monitoring showed mild improvement in glycemic patterns without any hypoglycemia.

[1]Department of Pediatrics, Division of Endocrinology and Diabetes, Helen Devos Children's Hospital, Spectrum Health, Michigan State University, Grand Rapids, Michigan. [2]Department of Pediatrics. [3]Department of Medicine, University of Minnesota, Minneapolis, Minnesota

DOI: 10.2337/9781580407663.37

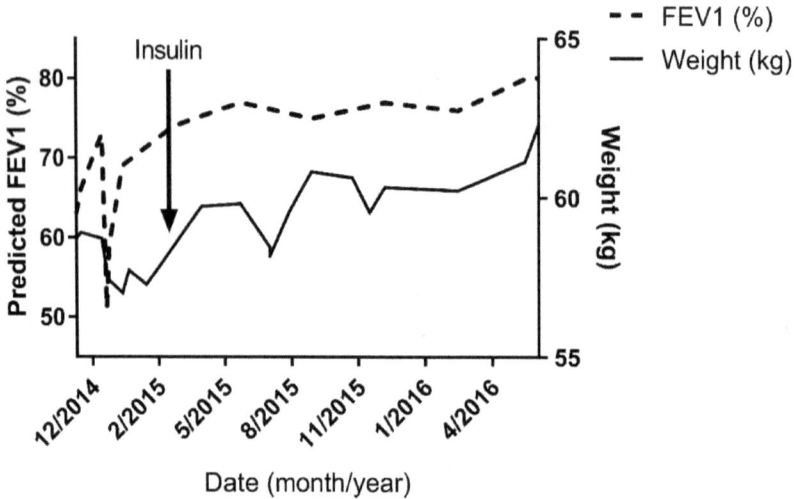

Figure 37.1—Change in pulmonary function and weight before and after initiation of insulin.

CFRD is the most common non-pulmonary complication associated with CF. The exact pathophysiology of CFRD is still unknown but is multifactorial. It is likely a combination of progressive pancreatic fibrosis leading to islet cell destruction, defective signaling related to CFTR, genetic factors, and eventually modest insulin resistance. Loss of first-phase insulin release is seen in early stages with progressive loss of second-phase insulin secretion. Irrespective of the exact mechanism of CFRD, the end result is functional insulinopenia, which results in catabolism. The prevalence of CFRD increases with age, with rates of >50% in adults who have CF. It is recommended that all patients with CF be screened annually by 2-h OGTT, starting at least by the age of 10 years.[1]

In other forms of diabetes, the impact of hyperglycemia on micro- and macrovascular disease drive morbidity and mortality. While CFRD has been associated with microvascular complications, these are generally mild compared to other types of diabetes, and macrovascular disease is rare in CFRD. CFRD is associated, however, with reduced survival; all-cause mortality in CF is increased by approximately sixfold in CF patients who develop CFRD, and death is almost universally related to exacerbation of CF pulmonary disease.

CFRD contributes to a catabolic state due to chronic insulinopenia. Low BMI and especially low lean body mass are associated with worse lung function and increased mortality in the CF population, and insulin insufficiency is associated with poor weight gain and increased protein catabolism. Fortunately, insulin therapy has been associated with improved weight gain and survival in CFRD, even in patients who, as in this case, have early CFRD without fasting hyperglycemia and with relatively normal glucose levels at home under usual living conditions. It is for this reason that insulin therapy is the only recommended treatment for CFRD, and it is recommended early in the course of the disease because protein catabolism is occurring well before the onset of clinical hyperglycemia.

CFRD may also contribute to worsening pulmonary function by promoting colonization of bacteria and fungi. The mechanism is thought to be due to increasing glucose concentration within mucosal secretions, providing a medium for growth of pathologic organisms. CFRD has been directly associated with worsening pulmonary function testing (FEV1), increase in frequency and severity of pulmonary exacerbations, increased hospitalization, and increased length of stay. In fact, CFRD should be suspected in a case where pulmonary function declines unexpectedly, such as in this case.[2]

Here are some takeaways from this case:

- The rationale for initiation of insulin therapy in CFRD differs from type 1 and type 2 diabetes.
- The primary rationale for insulin is to induce an anabolic state promoting macronutrient retention and weight gain. These factors are critical for survival in CF. Improvement in glycemic status is secondary, so relatively normal home glucose levels should not preclude instituting insulin therapy.
- Complications associated with CFRD include increased all-cause mortality, worsened pulmonary function, weight loss, and microvascular disease (not macrovascular disease).

COMMENTARY

CFRD is a frequent complication of CF that has a distinct clinical course from type 1 and type 2 diabetes. As the authors correctly pointed out, functional insulinopenia of CF results not only in hyperglycemia, but also in the profound inability to use nutrients to promote weight gain and suppression of catabolism. If we accept this premise, then it is logical that institution of early insulin therapy in patients with CRDF, even with minimal alterations in carbohydrate metabolism, is the most prudent course of action.

As illustrated by this case, both weight gain and improved pulmonary function followed initiation of insulin therapy. Whether the therapy should be started with a long-acting insulin or mealtime insulin, or both, is highly individualized depending on the clinical course of the disease.

Boris Draznin, MD, PhD

REFERENCES

1. Marshall B, Faro, Elbert A, et al. *2018 Patient Registry: Annual Data Report.* Bethesda, MD, Cystic Fibrosis Foundation, 2018

2. Granados A, Chan CL, Ode KL, Moheet A, Moran A, Holl R. Cystic fibrosis related diabetes: pathophysiology, screening and diagnosis. *J Cystic Fibros* 2019;18 (Suppl 2):S3–S9

Case 38

Cystic Fibrosis–Related Diabetes Case Series: Effects of the CF Transmembrane Conductance Regulator (CFTR) Modulator on Glycemic Control

Jagdeesh Ullal, MD,[1] Lina Merjaneh, MD,[2] Kara S. Hughan, MD,[3] and Andrea Kelly, MD, MSCE[4]

C ase 1 was a 20-year-old female with pancreatic insufficient cystic fibrosis (CF) (delF508/delF508), severe obstructive lung disease, cystic fibrosis–related diabetes (CFRD), malnutrition, depression, and nonadherence to treatment regimen. She experienced a significant decline in her clinical status with frequent hospitalizations about 2 years before initiating Trikafta. Her BMI declined from the 47th to <1st percentile and FEV_1%-predicted declined from 78 to 29. Her HbA_{1c} increased from 6.9 to 9.9%, and she had a diabetic ketoacidosis episode. Diabetes autoantibodies were negative.

Because of poor appetite and caloric intake, she was on relatively low doses of insulin before starting Trikafta (insulin glargine 4 units, insulin–to–carbohydrate ratio 1:30, and correction factor of 1 unit for every 180 mg/dL above 100 mg/dL; weight = 89.1 lb).

After starting Trikafta, her overall health and quality of life improved. FEV_1%-predicted improved from 26 to 48. However, diabetes control worsened significantly with a rise in HbA_{1c} within 1 month, from 9.9 to >14%, with symptoms of polyuria and polydipsia and weight loss of 5.1 kg. She was admitted with severe hyperglycemia (glucose 922 mg/dL), dehydration, and lethargy without diabetic ketoacidosis, which responded to intravenous hydration and intensive insulin treatment. She demonstrated improved appetite and significant increase in caloric intake while hospitalized, with a 22.3-lb weight increase within 1 month. She was discharged home on insulin glargine 10 units, insulin aspart–to–carbohydrate ratio of 1:14, and correction factor of 1 unit for every 60 mg/dL above 100 mg/dL. Subsequently, she was admitted twice with pulmonary exacerbations, severe

[1]University of Pittsburgh School of Medicine, University of Pittsburgh Medical Center, Center for Diabetes and Endocrinology, Pittsburgh, Pennsylvania. [2]Division of Endocrinology & Diabetes, Seattle Children's Hospital, Seattle, Washington. [3]Division of Endocrinology and Diabetes, University of Pittsburgh Medical Center Children's Hospital of Pittsburgh, University of Pittsburgh School of Medicine, Pittsburgh, Pennsylvania. [4]Children's Hospital of Philadelphia, University of Pennsylvania Perelman School of Medicine, Philadelphia, Pennsylvania

DOI: 10.2337/9781580407663.38

hyperglycemia, and weight loss. She was noncompliant with her outpatient insulin regimen. FEV_1%-predicted declined to 31%.

Worsening of her diabetes control after starting Trikafta was unexpected but could be explained by improved appetite and caloric intake and perhaps improved gastrointestinal function and absorption, which were offset by poor compliance with diabetes management. The lung function and overall health benefits of Trikafta were offset by severe hyperglycemia, which caused weight loss and fatigue and possibly increased her risk for infection and exacerbations.

Case 2 was a 48-year-old female with pancreatic-insufficient CF (delF508/delF508) who was diagnosed with CFRD at age 19 years during a hospitalization for pneumonia and glucocorticoid treatment, when her blood glucose concentrations were as high as 600 mg/dL. She had been treated with insulin over the subsequent 3 decades. In 2012, insulin pump therapy was initiated with a basal rate of 0.4 units/h (9.6 units/day), insulin-to-carbohydrate ratio of 1:20, and correction factor of 1 unit for every 60 mg/dL above 120 mg/dL. HbA_{1c} was 6.7% but underestimated her glucose control, since postprandial glucose levels were as high as 300 mg/dL.

Over the next 6 years, the same basal rate was maintained, but insulin-to-carbohydrate ratios varied: breakfast 1:16, lunch 1:20, and dinner 1:25. While her HbA_{1c} remained under 7% in 2018, her average glycemia was 191 ± 105 mg/dL on professional continuous glucose monitoring (CGM). In May 2019, her personal CGM helped improve her average glycemia to 150 ± 58 mg/dL, with only three episodes of hypoglycemia every 2 weeks. Two weeks after initiating Trikafta (January 2020), hypoglycemia became more frequent (up to six episodes every 2 weeks), and rapid descent of blood glucose required pump suspension several times a day to minimize hypoglycemia. Subsequent reduction of total basal dose from 7.8 to 3.9 units/day and relaxation of insulin-to-carbohydrate ratios to 1:25 addressed the recurrent hypoglycemia. No other medications had been introduced to explain the drastic decline in insulin requirements. Kidney function remained stable, and no signs of adrenal insufficiency (hypotension or anorexia) were present. The patient felt drastically better on Trikafta, and her glucose levels remained reasonably controlled with an HbA_{1c} of 5.7%.

Herein, we present two patients with CFRD who initiated the CF transmembrane conductance regulator (CFTR) modulator Trikafta, which resulted in drastic changes in glucose control.

CF is a multisystem disorder arising from mutations in the gene encoding CFTR. Diabetes is common in CF and, while sharing features with type 1 and type 2 diabetes, is a distinct form of diabetes and is categorized as pancreatogenous, or type 3c diabetes, arising from relative insulin deficiency due to pancreatic islet cell destruction.

CFTR regulates the chloride channel, and loss or dysfunction of chloride channels impairs chloride and sodium transport and leads to dehydration and desiccation of epithelial cells and mucous membranes. CFTR defects could directly or indirectly contribute to β-cell dysfunction and decreased insulin secretion. CFTR is highly expressed in the pancreatic ducts and is essential for proper duct function. Its loss from ductal epithelium may contribute to islet dysfunction in CF via paracrine mechanisms.[1] CFTR might have direct actions in β-cells, although this issue remains controversial.[2]

CFTR modulators are a class of drugs that improve synthesis, intracellular processing, and function of CFTR protein to address the primary defect in CF.[3] These drugs are classified as potentiators (ivacaftor), which increase CFTR channel opening, or as correctors (elexacaftor, lumacaftor, tezacaftor), which increase the amount of CFTR protein at the cell surface. A triple combination medication is highly effective in improving lung function in patients with the most common CFTR mutation, namely delF508. The CF community attained a significant milestone in therapeutic development when the U.S. Food and Drug Administration approved the triple combination pill elexacaftor-tezacaftor-ivacaftor (Trikafta) in October 2019 for patients with at least one delF508 mutation.

Reports of improved insulin secretion with CFTR modulators suggest potential mechanisms include *1)* CFTR-dependent islet-associated ductal function recovery, *2)* improved gut incretin function, and *3)* reduction of inflammation and insulin resistance of systemic illness.[4] We present two patients with CFRD who initiated the CFTR modulator Trikafta, which resulted in drastic changes in glucose control.

The pivotal trials of CFTR modulators have demonstrated a significant improvement in lung function and hold great potential in improving quality of life in people with CF.[5] The therapeutic effects of this drug class on other organ systems remain to be ascertained. A 2-year observational study (PROMISE; ClinicalTrials.gov: NCT04038047) was designed to address longer-term, multi-system outcomes. These case reports describe the effects of the newest CFTR modulator, Trikafta, on CFRD. Although these cases have very different glycemia outcomes, they highlight the need for close attention to glucose after initiation of CFTR modulator therapy and close collaboration between pulmonary and endocrine teams in the care of patients with CFRD.

COMMENTARY

These two cases illustrate not only tremendous advances in management of CF, but point out clinical problems arising from the use of these modulators in controlling glycemia in patients with CFRD. Individuals with CF require more energy to compensate for poor digestion and to fight lung infection. Their energy needs are estimated to be at least twice the needs of people without CF. Almost invariably, the diet of these patients is high in carbohydrates, especially in items containing simple sugars. Even though mealtime insulin calculated on the basis of insulin-to-carbohydrate ratio is a correct approach to manage their glycemia, the difficulties frequently lie in the timing mismatch between food intake and insulin administration. Most patients with CFRD do not adhere to a fixed food consumption schedule and instead may "graze" all day long. Many continuously sip sugar-containing beverages throughout the day, making insulin dosing difficult.

We do not know why in these two cases the same new CFTR modulator resulted in distinct glycemic changes, but the authors' conclusion about close monitoring of these patients is absolutely correct.

Boris Draznin, MD, PhD

REFERENCES

1. Bertelli E, Bendayan M. Association between endocrine pancreas and ductal system: more than an epiphenomenon of endocrine differentiation and development? *J Histochem Cytochem* 2005;53:1071–1086

2. Manderson Koivula FN, McClenaghan NH, Harper AGS, Kelly C. Correction to: Islet-intrinsic effects of CFTR mutation. *Diabetologia* 2017;60:2544

3. Grasemann H. CFTR modulator therapy for cystic fibrosis. *N Engl J Med* 2017;377:2085–2088

4. Kelly A, De Leon DD, Sheikh S, et al. Islet hormone and incretin secretion in cystic fibrosis after four months of ivacaftor therapy. *Am J Respir Crit Care Med* 2019;199:342–351

5. Keating D, Marigowda G, Burr L, et al. VX-445-tezacaftor-ivacaftor in patients with cystic fibrosis and one or two Phe508del alleles. *N Engl J Med* 2018;379:1612–1620

Part 8

Diabetes Management and Miscellaneous Cases

Case 39

Simplifying Insulin Therapy: Transitioning from Basal-Bolus Insulin Therapy to Basal Insulin With a Glucagon-Like Peptide-1 Receptor Analog (GLP-1RA)

Sevil Aliyeva, MD,[1] Pamela Schroeder, MD,PhD,[1] and Paul Sack, MD[1]

A 74-year-old African American woman with hypertension, hyperlipidemia, coronary artery disease, and recent stroke was seen for follow-up of type 2 diabetes complicated by retinopathy and peripheral neuropathy. She was diagnosed with type 2 diabetes at age 56 years and was treated with metformin; subsequently, sitagliptin was added. For the past 7 years, she has been on multiple daily insulin (MDI) injections with glargine 30 units daily and lispro 10 units with meals. However, this regimen has been challenging to her, since she frequently eats without taking mealtime insulin, which leads to hyperglycemia. She also frequently has fasting and postprandial hypoglycemia, based on continuous glucose monitoring. Her type 2 diabetes is uncontrolled with recent HbA$_{1c}$ of 12%.

Type 2 diabetes is a chronic, progressive disease characterized by multiple defects in glucose metabolism, including insulin resistance in muscle, liver, and adipocytes; progressive β-cell failure; hyperglucagonemia; impaired incretin effect; and increased glucose reabsorption in the kidneys. β-Cell failure progresses at a rate of ~4% per year, which requires progressive escalation of medications to insulin therapy to achieve glycemic control.[1,2]

The American Diabetes Association (ADA) type 2 diabetes medical management algorithm recommends metformin initially, but options such as glucagon-like peptide-1 receptor agonists (GLP-1RAs) and oral hypoglycemic agents are available if adequate control is not obtained. Insulin is recommended as the preferred agent in patients with symptomatic hyperglycemia, HbA$_{1c}$ >10%, or glucose >300 mg/dL. Ultimately, these patients may progress to MDI therapy.[3]

Basal-bolus insulin therapy has traditionally been considered to be the best way to manage uncontrolled type 2 diabetes, but this may not actually be needed for many patients with the advent of GLP-1RAs. MDI therapy has many challenges including hypoglycemia, weight gain, poor adherence, and cost. Although the ADA algorithm is clear on how to titrate up the noninsulin and insulin therapies, there are no evidence-based guidelines on deescalating

[1]Division of Endocrinology, Medstar Union Memorial Hospital, Baltimore, Maryland

DOI: 10.2337/9781580407663.39

insulin therapy by adding noninsulin medications. GLP-1RAs are potential candidates to use when attempting to decrease or replace insulin in patients with type 2 diabetes failing MDI.

Because our patient was having significant challenges with MDI therapy, we decided to add the weekly GLP-1RA semaglutide, titrating it to the maximum dose over 8 weeks. It was well tolerated, and she lost 6.6 lb over 5 months. Her appetite decreased. As the semaglutide was increased, her insulin dose was reduced to avoid hypoglycemia. Both basal and mealtime insulins were decreased by 20% with each dose escalation of semaglutide. Patient satisfaction increased with discontinuation of mealtime insulin and a simplified regimen of glargine 16 units daily and semaglutide 1 mg weekly. Her HbA$_{1c}$ has dropped to 7.3% with blood glucose levels of 100–140 mg/dL fasting and 100–160 mg/dL postprandially without hypoglycemia.

GLP-1RAs are important agents for the management of type 2 diabetes because of their multifactorial mechanism of action. They stimulate the β-cells of the pancreas to produce insulin in a glucose-dependent fashion and reduce the postprandial rise in glucagon after meals, which results in less glucose output from the liver. This dual action results in glucose lowering. GLP-1RAs also slow gastric emptying, which decreases the rate of absorption of glucose. Additionally, these medications act centrally to promote satiety. In randomized controlled trials, the main reason for drug discontinuation was gastrointestinal (GI) side effects.

Adding GLP-1RAs to basal insulin can ameliorate side effects of basal insulin including hypoglycemia and weight gain. Because of the β-cell–dependent primary mechanism of action of GLP-1RAs, its efficacy is questioned in patients with long-standing diabetes or in patients who have been on basal-bolus therapy for years. Anecdotally, however, many patients with long-standing diabetes respond well to these medications.

In patients with type 2 diabetes, combination therapy with GLP-1RA and insulin proved to be as effective as MDI in terms of HbA$_{1c}$, while leading to a significant weight loss, reduced risk of hypoglycemia, and lower insulin doses. Because the addition of GLP-1RA could exert the same glucose-lowering effects of up to 60 IU/day of insulin, patients on MDI therapy could potentially benefit from changing to GLP-1RA/insulin regimens.[3]

In the AWARD-9 (Assessment of Weekly Administration of Dulaglutide in Diabetes-9) and AWARD-4 trials, dulaglutide 1.5 mg subcutaneously weekly demonstrated superiority versus placebo when added to titrated insulin glargine with a change in HbA$_{1c}$ from baseline (–1.44 vs. –0.67% at 26 weeks). This dose also demonstrated superiority versus insulin glargine when combined with insulin lispro three times daily with a change in HbA$_{1c}$ from baseline (–1.64 vs. –1.41% at 26 weeks), respectively. These findings were observed in patients age >65 years, with poorly controlled type 2 diabetes with HbA$_{1c}$ level >9% and diabetes duration >10 years.[4] Dulaglutide has been approved for use in combination with basal and/or prandial insulin.

The MDI Liraglutide Trial studied MDI therapy with either liraglutide or placebo in overweight and obese patients with long-standing type 2 diabetes and HbA$_{1c}$ of 7.5–11.5%. HbA$_{1c}$ level was reduced by 1.1% ($P < 0.001$), and weight was reduced by 3.8 kg ($P < 0.001$) in participants treated with liraglutide compared with control subjects. Better glycemic control was obtained despite a lowering of insulin doses by an average of 15.8 units in the liraglutide group compared with placebo at 24 weeks.[5]

Potential cardiovascular benefit is also a reason to consider the addition of a GLP-1RA. Multiple large randomized controlled trials have reported significant reductions in cardiovascular events in type 2 diabetes patients treated with GLP-1RAs (liraglutide [LEADER], semaglutide [SUSTAIN-6], dulaglutide [REWIND], lixisenatide [ELIXA], oral semaglutide [PIONEER], and exenatide [EXCEL]).[6] Thus, a practical extension of these results to clinical practice is highlighted in the ADA guidelines. GLP-1RAs are recommended as the preferred second-line treatment option (after metformin) in patients with T2D and established atherosclerotic cardiovascular disease (ASCVD) or indicators of high ASCVD risk.[6]

We conclude that based on the few randomized controlled trials and case reports, patients with partially preserved insulin secretion may benefit from changing MDI therapy to simpler treatments with the potential for improved glycemic control, less hypoglycemia, decrease in weight, and cardiovascular risk reduction. Further randomized clinical trials are needed to elucidate the best way to safely add GLP-1RAs to MDI therapy.

COMMENTARY

I am delighted to see how creatively our colleagues are trying to find better and simplified ways of controlling diabetes in their patients. Using GLP-1RAs as an alternative approach to mealtime insulin has gained wide acceptance. This case lends additional support to this strategy and provides a short but important review of the clinical trials relevant to this approach.

Using GLP-1RAs along with basal insulin does indeed simplify the therapeutic regimen. While more randomized clinical trials are needed to provide better guidelines for this approach, the cardiovascular benefits of GLP-1RAs, which are so critically important for patients with type 2 diabetes, make this class of drugs ideal for many patients with type 2 diabetes.

Boris Draznin, MD, PhD

REFERENCES

1. DeFronzo RA. From the triumvirate to the ominous octet: a new paradigm for the treatment of type 2 diabetes mellitus. *Diabetes* 2009;58:773–795

2. U.K. Prospective Diabetes Study Group. U.K. Prospective Diabetes Study 16. Overview of 6 years' therapy of type II diabetes: a progressive disease. *Diabetes* 1995;44:1249–1258

3. American Diabetes Association. 9. Pharmacologic approaches to glycemic treatment: *Standards of Medical Care in Diabetes—2020. Diabetes Care* 2020;43 (Suppl. 1):S98–S110

4. KM Pantalone. Dulaglutide 1.5 mg as an add-on option for patients uncontrolled on insulin: subgroup analysis by age, duration of diabetes and baseline glycated hemoglobin concentration. *Diabetes Obes Metab* 2018;20:1461–1469

5. Lind M. Liraglutide in people treated for type 2 diabetes with multiple daily insulin injections: randomized clinical trial (MDI Liraglutide trial). *BMJ* 2015;351:h5364

6. Kristensen SL. Cardiovascular, mortality, and kidney outcomes with GLP-1 receptor agonists in patients with type 2 diabetes: a systematic review and meta-analysis of cardiovascular outcome trials. *Lancet* 2019;7:776–785

Case 40

Simplification of Insulin Regimen Improves Glycemic Control in Elderly Patients With Type 2 Diabetes

Maria Gracia Luzuriaga, MD,[1] and Rajesh Garg, MD[1]

Case 1 was a 72-year-old female with type 2 diabetes who presented to our clinic to optimize glycemic control. The patient had a history of end-stage renal disease (ESRD) related to prolonged hypertension, and she had received a kidney transplant about 5 years before presentation. The patient was diagnosed with diabetes 3 years prior (2 years after renal transplant) and was started on insulin soon after the diagnosis. On our initial evaluation, she had an HbA$_{1c}$ of 10.0%. No other significant problems were detected and she reported no hypoglycemia. Her kidney function revealed an eGFR of 60 mL/min/1.73 m^2. She was taking tacrolimus and mycophenolate as anti-rejection therapy. Her insulin regimen consisted of 36 units insulin glargine at bedtime and 12 units insulin lispro before every meal. She was also monitoring her blood glucose level 2–4 times daily at home. The patient was retired, but independent in her daily activities, and her cognition was intact. She claimed to be following the regimen but admitted to forgetting to take insulin at times.

After discussion, the patient was switched to once-daily injection of 50 units insulin glargine in the morning and advised to stop her premeal insulin. She was advised to monitor her blood glucose twice a day. Her glycemic control improved significantly at 3 months, with an HbA$_{1c}$ of 7.8%. One year later, the patient continues on insulin glargine 60 units daily, and her most recent HbA$_{1c}$ was 6.7%. She has not reported any episodes of symptomatic hypoglycemia or blood glucose levels <54 mg/dL.

Case 2 was a 71-year-old male with type 2 diabetes who presented to our clinic to optimize glycemic control. The patient had multiple comorbidities including hypertension, heart failure secondary to ischemic cardiomyopathy, Paget's disease of the bone, and severe osteoarthritis. The patient was diagnosed with diabetes >30 years ago. He was treated with noninsulin hypoglycemic agents for the initial ~20 years and then transitioned to insulin. His diabetes control had been poor for many years, and the most recent HbA$_{1c}$ was 12.8%. His treatment regimen included 46 units insulin detemir at bedtime and 12 units insulin lispro before every meal. He

[1]Division of Endocrinology, Diabetes, and Metabolism, University of Miami, Miller School of Medicine, Miami, Florida

DOI: 10.2337/9781580407663.40

was monitoring his blood glucose level 3–4 times a day and reported occasional episodes of hypoglycemia. The patient did not have stable housing; therefore, he had limited access to proper insulin storage.

The patient was transitioned to 40 units insulin glargine twice daily and was advised to monitor his blood glucose twice a day. A sodium–glucose cotransporter 2 (SGLT2) inhibitor drug was prescribed but rejected by his insurance company. The patient was followed regularly in the clinic, and his insulin dose was adjusted. His glycemic control improved with a follow-up HbA_{1c} of 9.9% after 3 months. The patient was transitioned later to once-daily injection of insulin glargine. After 2 years, his HbA_{1c} was 8.0% on 70 units insulin glargine daily, without hypoglycemia.

The prevalence of type 2 diabetes has been increasing over time, especially in the older age-groups. Many elderly patients (>65 years of age) with type 2 diabetes have other comorbidities like heart disease, renal insufficiency, cognitive impairment, and lack of social support.[1] They also have an increased risk of hypoglycemia. Taking these factors into consideration, the American Diabetes Association (ADA) recommends an HbA_{1c} goal <7.5% in the elderly patients in overall good health and <8.5% in patients with multiple comorbidities.[1] Individualized treatment plans using simple medication regimens with low potential for hypoglycemia are recommended.[1]

However, even for relatively relaxed glycemic goals, insulin treatment is often necessary for many elderly patients because they are poor candidates for noninsulin antidiabetic agents.[2] Currently, the majority of elderly patients on insulin receive basal-bolus insulin therapy that includes four injections daily. This insulin regimen is often confusing and hard to manage. Simplification of insulin regimen may improve glycemic control in these patients besides improving their quality of life.[3]

Our two cases demonstrate that simplification of insulin regimen improves glycemic control in elderly patients when basal-bolus insulin regimen is failing and/or imposing undue treatment burden. The cases presented in this report are not unique. However, our purpose is to highlight an extremely important clinical strategy that is rarely used in practice. Most physicians tend to either increase the insulin doses or add a correctional insulin scale when target HbA_{1c} is not achieved. However, as demonstrated by the above cases, the root cause of problem is failure to follow the complex treatment regimen. Therefore, backing off from a complex insulin regimen often improves HbA_{1c}, decreases the risk of hypoglycemia, and improves quality of life.

The major goal of managing type 2 diabetes is to achieve an appropriate reduction in glucose levels to minimize the risk of complications. A patient's life expectancy and risk of developing complications of diabetes are key factors in selecting a glycemic target. Adverse effects of the treatment regimen itself must also be prevented. Older adults deserve an individualized approach that should take into consideration their medical, psychological, functional, and social domains. Patients who are expected to live long enough to benefit from long-term intensive diabetes management, who have a good cognitive and physical function, and who choose to do so via shared decision-making may be treated using therapeutic interventions and goals similar to those for younger adults with diabetes.[1] However, a large majority of elderly patients might benefit from a simplified insulin regimen that provides an acceptable glycemic control. Simplification of complex insulin therapy and de-intensification of treatment is recommended in older patients in the ADA standards of clinical care.[1] However, this recommendation is often ignored, as shown by previous studies.[4,5] We suggest that the insulin regimen should be periodically reevaluated and simplified when a complex regimen is failing in an elderly patient.

COMMENTARY

Individualization of glycemic targets and a shared decision-making process to reach these targets are rapidly becoming the standard approach to treatment of diabetes. More than in any other situation, this approach is gaining acceptance in treatment of elderly patients and individuals with various significant comorbidities. With improved life expectancy that takes us into the mid-80s, the previous definition of elderly (>65 years of age) will probably need to be revised. There are many healthy adults who keep their excellent health and vigor way beyond age 65 years. Among those individuals are also people with diabetes who do not have any other medical conditions and have minimal or no complications of diabetes. These patients would benefit from better glycemic control, as do younger patients with diabetes.

On the other hand, others might have many more medical problems or a combination of medical and socioeconomic problems. These individuals would benefit from individualized, more relaxed targets that can be safely achieved by simplifying their therapeutic regimen. The two cases presented by Drs. Luzuriaga and Garg provide excellent illustration of this approach. Both patients were switched from basal-bolus insulin regimens to basal insulin, with great improvement in glycemic control.

There is nothing wrong with this approach as long as a careful and close follow-up plan is in place. Even though the current basal-only therapy appears to be working now, there is no guarantee it will continue working in the future. Therapy will likely have to be adjusted to reinstitute mealtime insulin or to add glucagon-like peptide-1 (GLP-1) receptor agonist or SGLT2 inhibitors, for example. One also has to be extremely careful not to over-insulinize a patient with too much basal insulin, which can lead to significant glycemic variability and hypoglycemia. Unfortunately, this latter scenario is far too common in the real world.

Overall, simplification of insulin regimen is a good thing in vulnerable populations. But always remember, "First Do No Harm" ("Primum Non Nocere"), since vigilance and ability to adjust must remain our guiding principles.

Boris Draznin, MD, PhD

REFERENCES

1. American Diabetes Association. 12. Older adults: *Standards of Medical Care in Diabetes—2020. Diabetes Care* 2020:43(Suppl. 1):S152–S162

2. Kirkman MS, Briscoe VJ, Clark N, et al. Diabetes in older adults. *Diabetes Care* 2012;35:2650–2664

3. Munshi MN, Slyne C, Segal AR, Saul N, Lyons C, Weigner K. Simplification of insulin regimen in older adults and risk of hypoglycemia. *JAMA Intern Med* 2016;176:1023–1025

4. Pirela DV, Garg R. De-intensification of diabetes treatment in elderly patients with type 2 diabetes mellitus. *Endocr Pract* 2019;25:1317–1322

5. Weiner JZ, Gopalan A, Mishra P, et al. Use and discontinuation of insulin treatment among adults aged 75 to 79 years with type 2 diabetes. *JAMA Intern Med* 2019;179:1633–1641

Case 41

Effects of Glucagon-Like Peptide-1 Receptor Agonist (GLP-1RA) in an Individual With Type 2 Diabetes on High-Dose Insulin Therapy

Basem M. Mishriky, MD,[1] Doyle M. Cummings, PharmD, FCP, FCCP,[2] and Carlos E. Mendez, MD[3]

The patient is a 55-year-old male with a history of type 2 diabetes, coronary artery disease (CAD), and class III obesity who was evaluated in the diabetes clinic. His diabetes regimen included metformin XR 2 g daily, insulin glargine 80 units daily, and insulin lispro 40 units before meals. His HbA$_{1c}$ was 8.4%, weight 313.7 lb, BMI 40.29 kg/m^2, and insulin-to-weight ratio 1.4 units/kg/daily.

Given his established history of CAD, initiating a glucagon-like peptide-1 receptor agonist (GLP-1RA) was discussed with him, and subcutaneous semaglutide 0.25 mg once weekly with the recommended fixed-dose escalation was started. Since his HbA$_{1c}$ was >8.0%, his insulin doses were not reduced initially and metformin was continued; however, he was educated to consider self-reduction of premeal insulin doses in the event of developing hypoglycemia or by 10–15% if glycemic targets (defined as a fasting and premeal glucose measurement between 80 and 130 mg/dL) were consistently achieved. He was also prescribed continuous glucose monitoring (CGM).

Within 2 weeks after the initiation of semaglutide, his glycemic targets were achieved. He then self-reduced insulin lispro by 10–15% weekly until he was seen by his primary care provider. Approximately 2 months later, his HbA$_{1c}$ was 5.5%, and the insulin glargine dose was reduced by 30%. When the patient was seen again in the diabetes clinic, his CGM data showed time in range (TIR) of 85% with an average glucose of 102 mg/dL. To facilitate further reduction in his insulin, the semaglutide dose was titrated to 1 mg weekly for maximum benefit. Given that he achieved glycemic targets and his semaglutide dose had been increased, his basal and mealtime insulin doses were reduced by 40%. He returned to clinic 1 month later, and his CGM download showed a continued TIR of 84%. Insulin lispro was discontinued at that time and insulin glargine was gradually discontinued over the next 3 months. Approximately 10 months after the initiation

[1]Department of Internal Medicine. [2]Department of Family Medicine, East Carolina University, Greenville, North Carolina. [3]Division of Diabetes and Endocrinology, Froedtert and Medical College of Wisconsin, Milwaukee, Wisconsin

DOI: 10.2337/9781580407663.41

of semaglutide, the patient was completely off insulin, remaining on subcutaneous semaglutide and metformin. His HbA_{1c} improved to 5.6%, and his BMI was reduced to 35.4 kg/m^2, representing a 37.5-lb weight loss.

The case represents an individual with type 2 diabetes who, on initial evaluation, had evidence of obesity-related insulin resistance requiring high-dose insulin. Given his history of CAD, a discussion to add noninsulin medication with cardiovascular benefits was initiated with the patient. Subcutaneous semaglutide was added to his regimen of metformin and high-dose insulin, resulting in better glycemic control without severe hypoglycemia. Ten months after the initiation of subcutaneous semaglutide, he lost 37.5 lb and insulin was discontinued.

Type 2 diabetes is a progressive disease and many patients might require intensification of their regimen by adding and titrating insulin. However, individuals with type 2 diabetes and obesity are insulin resistant and hyperinsulinemic.[1] Exogenous insulin can exaggerate hyperinsulinemia, promote additional weight gain, and occasionally cause hypoglycemia.

Whereas there are clear recommendations on adding noninsulin medications with evidence of cardiovascular benefit when metformin alone fails, there are few recommendations available regarding the initiation of noninsulin medications in patients who are already on high-dose insulin. The addition of GLP-1RA to individuals with type 2 diabetes on high-dose insulin poses some risk of hypoglycemia, but it has been shown to be safe and effective.[2-4] Lane et al.[3] investigated the addition of liraglutide to individuals on >100 units/day of insulin. Baseline HbA_{1c} was used to determine if insulin dose adjustment was indicated, using the following guideline: HbA_{1c} <7.0% (50% reduction in mealtime insulin and 25% reduction in basal insulin), HbA_{1c} 7.1–8.0% (25% reduction in both basal and mealtime insulin), and HbA_{1c} >8.0% (no reduction in insulin). Vanderheiden et al.,[4] investigating the addition of liraglutide to individuals on >1.5 units/kg/day insulin, did not reduce insulin doses at baseline if HbA_{1c} was >8.0% but reduced insulin doses by 20% if HbA_{1c} was <8.0%. Following the initiation of liraglutide, insulin doses were adjusted by 10–20% if finger-stick blood glucose readings revealed hypoglycemia and by 30% if severe hypoglycemia was evident. Both trials concluded that there was a greater HbA_{1c} reduction and more weight loss with liraglutide at 6 months.

Although it is generally safe to add GLP-1RA to high-dose insulin in individuals with T2D and insulin resistance, we recommend a cautious approach to avoid hypoglycemia. When adding the GLP-1RA, if the baseline HbA_{1c} is <8.0%, we suggest at least a 20% reduction in all insulin doses. If the baseline HbA_{1c} is >8.0% and there is no history of severe hypoglycemia, no reduction in insulin doses may be required, provided that the patient is willing and able to perform self-reduction of insulin if hypoglycemia were to occur. It may also be helpful to provide the patient with a recommended "protocol" for dosage adjustment.

Once GLP-1RA is added to high-dose insulin, it is suggested to consider regular telephone contact and to reevaluate the patient in 2–4 weeks. In the absence of hypoglycemia, patients may be followed in the office in 4–12 weeks depending on their individual risk for developing hypoglycemia. It is our suggestion that, if patients consistently achieve glycemic targets (defined as premeal glucose measurements of 80–130 mg/dL), all insulin doses should be reduced by at least 10% to proactively prevent hypoglycemia.

However, adding GLP-1RA to high-dose insulin is not without risk. Hypoglycemia remains an important risk, especially in patients who cannot self-titrate insulin doses. This process may require even more frequent follow-up visits, monitoring, and education. CGM can be extremely helpful during this process.

In summary, we present a case and discussion that focus on a relatively common patient scenario in primary care practice, for which limited clinical guidance is available. Specifically, we have illustrated an approach to safely initiating GLP-1RA therapy in individuals with type 2 diabetes, obesity, and insulin resistance who are already receiving high-dose insulin therapy. With careful monitoring and patient self-management training, GLP-1RA treatment can be successfully initiated, insulin therapy tapered and discontinued, glycemic control and BMI improved, and severe hypoglycemia avoided. We recommend using CGM whenever possible to facilitate glycemic monitoring and frequent telephone and office contacts with these patients.

DISCLOSURE

This information was adapted with permission from Wolters Kluwer Health, Inc.[5]

COMMENTARY

The most efficacious ways of using add-on therapy in type 2 diabetes patients is still the subject of research and clinical trials. With the entry of GLP-1RAs and sodium–glucose cotransporter 2 (SGLT2) inhibitors into the clinical arena, these two classes of medications have rapidly become favorite second-line (and, in some cases, first-line) medications when metformin in combination with lifestyle changes is not sufficient to produce good glycemic control. However, there were few studies and practically no guidelines as to how to add these medications to patients who are already on insulin, especially on high doses of insulin.

In this case, the authors describe successful addition of a GLP-1RA to metformin and high-dose insulin therapy while avoiding hypoglycemia and down-titrating insulin.

There are a few important points of this case. First is that a combination of insulin and GLP-1RA is a powerful combination to achieve desired glycemic control in patients with type 2 diabetes. It is prudent to reduce the doses of insulin while initiating this combination. Second is that patient education and the ability to self-titrate insulin doses are critically important to avoid hypoglycemia. However, this step is not easy to achieve in primary care practice because few, if any, practices can provide diabetes education. Community resources must therefore be used.

The third point is the importance of close follow-up when starting this combination to avoid untoward effects. With appropriate precautions and close follow-up, adding a GLP-1RA to insulin is an effective and safe approach to achieving good glycemic control in type 2 diabetes patients in primary care practices.

Boris Draznin, MD, PhD

REFERENCES

1. Nolan CJ, Ruderman NB, Kahn SE, Pedersen O, Prentki M. Insulin resistance as a physiological defense against metabolic stress: implications for the management of subsets of type 2 diabetes. *Diabetes* 2015;64:673–686

2. Lane W, Weinrib S, Rappaport J. The effect of liraglutide added to U-500 insulin in patients with type 2 diabetes and high insulin requirements. *Diabetes Technol Ther* 2011;13:592–595

3. Lane W, Weinrib S, Rappaport J, Hale C. The effect of addition of liraglutide to high-dose intensive insulin therapy: a randomized prospective trial. *Diabetes Obes Metab* 2014;16:827–832

4. Vanderheiden A, Harrison L, Warshauer J, Li X, Adams-Huet B, Lingvay I. Effect of adding liraglutide vs placebo to a high-dose insulin regimen in patients with type 2 diabetes: a randomized clinical trial. *JAMA Intern Med* 2016;176:939–947

5. Mishriky BM, Cummings DM, Mendez C, Patil SP, Powell JR. Transitioning to non-insulin therapy in a patient receiving high dose insulin. *J Am Assoc Nurse Pract* 2020;32:469–475

Case 42

Transient Severe Insulin Resistance in COVID-19 and Prediabetes

R. Matthew Hawkins, PA-C,[1] Whitney Adair, PA-C,[1] Joanna Gibbs, PA-C,[1] Jennifer Vinh, AGCNS-BC,[1] and Cecilia C. Low Wang, MD[1]

A 40-year-old woman presented with 6 days of worsening dyspnea. She had a history of prediabetes, hypertension, chronic hypoxic respiratory insufficiency, and severe obesity with a BMI of 69 kg/m². She was diagnosed with coronavirus disease 2019 (COVID-19) infection and admitted to the hospital. Over the first 7 days of hospitalization, her clinical course worsened. She was transferred to the intensive care unit with acute respiratory distress syndrome, intubated, and enteral feeding was initiated. Despite her critical illness, she remained euglycemic and did not require insulin therapy during this time, with blood glucose (BG) levels ranging from 91–162 mg/dL. On hospital days 9 and 10, the patient became progressively hyperglycemic and was diagnosed with ventilator-assisted pneumonia. She was started on an intravenous infusion of regular insulin. She demonstrated a marked increase in insulin needs without changes in her enteral feeding regimen, vasopressors, or the addition of glucocorticoid. On day 10, subcutaneous glargine was added to her insulin regimen. Over days 12–21, the patient continued to receive very high total daily doses (TDDs) of insulin, ranging from 572 to 912 units. On day 20, her subcutaneous insulin was changed from glargine to 70/30 insulin (Figure 42.1).

Hyperglycemia in hospitalized patients results from exaggerated counter-regulatory hormone response to medical and surgical stressors in patients with or without preexisting diabetes.

Numerous studies have established the relationship between elevated glucose levels and adverse clinical outcomes in critically ill patients, including Umpierrez et al. in 2002.[1] This phenomenon has also been observed and reported in patients with COVID-19 infection. Persistent hyperglycemia in COVID-19 patients is associated with a more than fourfold increase in mortality in patients with or without preexisting diabetes.[2] Although a causative relationship between elevated glucose and mortality has not been definitively established, the treatment of persistent hyperglycemia in hospitalized patients is generally accepted as standard of care.[3]

In our experience working with hospitalized patients infected with SARS-CoV-2, the insulin resistance and high insulin requirements exhibited

[1]University of Colorado School of Medicine, Aurora, Colorado

DOI: 10.2337/9781580407663.42

by this patient are not unique, and this case presentation represents a trend seen in multiple patients. What makes this patient's situation unique is the absence of preexisting diabetes and the absence of glucocorticoids during her hospitalization. Despite a lack of diabetes history, this patient exhibited severe hyperglycemia and insulin resistance similar to that which is observed in patients with coexisting diabetes and COVID-19 infection. This stress hyperglycemia appeared to be associated with the severity of her respiratory disease and was not reflected in inflammatory biomarkers such as C-reactive protein and d-dimer, or other factors such as carbohydrate content or route of administration of her nutrition. While the patient had predisposing risk factors for stress hyperglycemia, including prediabetes and severe obesity, the degree of insulin resistance she experienced was striking.

On hospital day 22, the patient's insulin needs decreased as suddenly as they rose, and the intravenous insulin was discontinued. The patient's pulmonary status improved, and she was weaned off the ventilator on day 23. Her BG remained below 150 mg/dL during this time without any need for insulin. This trend continued from days 24–30, with the patient receiving only 1 unit of insulin during this time period.

Another interesting observation in this case is the transient nature of her hyperglycemia and insulin resistance. The increase in insulin requirements in this patient was rapid and extreme. Her TDD of insulin increased from 0 to 3.6 units/kg within 4 days, reaching a maximum TDD of 5.7 units/kg. Equally notable was the dramatic decrease in this patient's insulin requirements over 24 h coinciding with significant clinical improvement. This result underscores the importance of close monitoring of glucose with appropriate adjustment of insulin dosing when treating stress hyperglycemia in patients with COVID-19.

One question raised by this patient's hospital course is whether her high insulin doses represent true demand or whether they were partially artifactual. Saturation of insulin receptors occurs at a certain threshold of insulin concentration[4] and may account for her high insulin doses. However, despite receptor saturation, it is likely that the severity of the respiratory infection and critical illness caused by SARS-CoV-2 in this patient with severe obesity and prediabetes is sufficient to explain the degree of insulin resistance, impairment in insulin production, and subsequent insulin requirements.

Our case presentation highlights the importance of recognizing prediabetes in patients with COVID-19. Stress hyperglycemia should serve as a red flag for both patients and clinicians, since the hazard ratio for developing subsequent diabetes is almost twofold after an episode of stress hyperglycemia, even after adjustment for age and severity of illness.[5] This case illustrates how insulin resistance, BG, and insulin needs may vary dramatically over the course of hospitalization in patients with COVID-19 infection. It is prudent for providers caring for patients with prediabetes to continue close BG monitoring throughout the hospitalization, especially during clinical condition or nutritional changes.

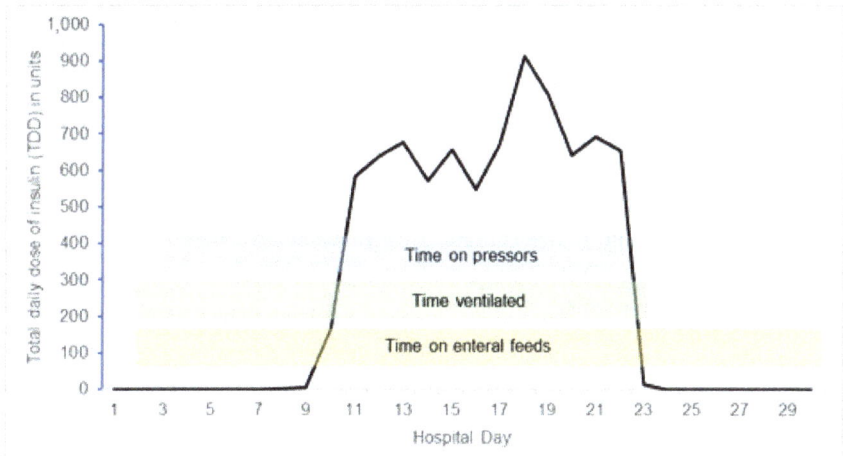

Figure 42.1—TDD of insulin trends over duration of admission.

COMMENTARY

Obesity and diabetes are among the important risk factors for unfavorable outcomes in patients with COVID-19 infection. The patient in this presentation is morbidly obese (BMI >68 kg/m²) and has prediabetes by history. It is not surprising that during severe acute illness her BG levels became elevated. Stress hyperglycemia is a common condition among hospitalized patients and is known to negatively affect outcomes, including mortality. Hyperglycemia can be further augmented by the use of medications such as pressors and steroids, and enteral nutrition. What is interesting is that, in this case, hyperglycemia appeared rapidly on day 9 of hospitalization, required extremely high doses of insulin, and disappeared equally rapidly within a day or two, on days 22–23. While an explanation for this unusual course of hyperglycemia is still lacking, the authors correctly indicate vigilance in following glycemia in COVID-19 patients and careful titration of insulin doses upwards and downwards to avoid further complications of glycemic management.

Boris Draznin, MD, PhD

REFERENCES

1. Umpierrez GE, Isaacs SD, Bazargan N, You X, Thaler LM, Kitabchi AE. Hyperglycemia: an independent marker of in-hospital mortality in patients with undiagnosed diabetes. *J Clin Endocrinol Metab* 2002;87:978–982

2. Bode B, Garrett V, Messler J, et al. Glycemic characteristics and clinical outcomes of COVID-19 patients hospitalized in the United States. *J Diabetes Sci Technol* 2020;14:813–821

3. American Diabetes Association. 15. Diabetes care in the hospital: *Standards of Medical Care in Diabetes—2020. Diabetes Care* 2020;43(Suppl. 1):S193–S202

4. Prigeon RL, Røder ME, Porte D Jr, Kahn SE. The effect of insulin dose on the measurement of insulin sensitivity by the minimal model technique: evidence for saturable insulin transport in humans. *J Clin Invest* 1996;97:501–507

5. Plummer MP, Finnis ME, Phillips LK, et al. Stress-induced hyperglycemia and the subsequent risk of type 2 diabetes in survivors of critical illness. *PLoS One* 2016;11:e0165923

Nondiabetic Renal Disease in Type 1 Diabetes: When to Consider a Renal Biopsy

Rong Mei Zhang, MD,[1] Ritika Puri, MD,[2] Tingting Li, MD,[3] and Janet B. McGill, MD[1]

Case 1 was a 33-year-old male with type 1 diabetes since age 6 years and hypothyroidism due to Hashimoto's thyroiditis; the patient missed annual labs for 2 years. He used continuous subcutaneous insulin infusion (CSII) and had achieved an HbA_{1c} level of <7% for several years. He previously took quinapril for microalbuminuria, but discontinued it and had undetectable microalbuminuria 2 years prior. He did not have retinopathy or neuropathy. In 2018, he complained of ankle swelling, his blood pressure was elevated at 172/96 mmHg, and his urine albumin-to-creatinine ratio (ACR) was 1,932 µg/mg. He was started on lisinopril 20 mg and further investigation was undertaken.

Laboratory evaluation showed normal serum creatinine of 0.94 mg/dL, low serum albumin of 2.5 g/dL, and high LDL of 140 mg/dL. Tests for hepatitis B and C and HIV were negative. ANA screen, anti-DsDNA antibody, SSA and SSB, anti-Smith antibody, anti-RNP antibody, UPEP, and anti-GBM antibody were negative. Urine protein-to-creatinine ratio increased to 5,124 mg/24 h. Urinalysis was positive for protein 3+, blood 1+, red blood cells (RBCs) 3–10 cells/hpf, and hyaline casts 1–3/hpf.

Because of well-controlled diabetes without retinopathy, the presence of microscopic hematuria, and nephrotic-range proteinuria, the patient underwent a renal biopsy. Pathology showed focal segmental glomerulosclerosis (FSGS) with mesangial staining for IgA (2+). Scattered mesangial electron dense deposits and podocyte foot process effacement was noted on electron microscopy, consistent with IgA diabetic kidney disease with FSGS, tip variant (Figure 43.1*A* and *B*). Diabetic kidney disease was not seen.

The patient was treated with high-dose prednisone, lisinopril, and furosemide. Despite an initial partial response, eventually proteinuria worsened to >10 g/day, prompting treatment with tacrolimus. Proteinuria improved and kidney function remained stable on this regimen.

Case 2 was a 38-year-old male with type 1 diabetes, hypertension, hyperlipidemia, and selective IgM deficiency who had significant albuminuria on

[1]Division of Endocrinology, Metabolism, and Lipid Research, Washington University School of Medicine, St. Louis, Missouri; [2]Division of Endocrinology, University of Nebraska Medical Center, Omaha, Nebraska; and [3]Division of Nephrology, Washington University School of Medicine, St. Louis, Missouri

DOI: 10.2337/9781580407663.43

routine screening. Type 1 diabetes was diagnosed at age 12 years and was well controlled with HbA_{1c} levels ranging from 6–7.5%. He managed his diabetes with continuous subcutaneous insulin infusion (CSII) along with a continuous glucose monitor and took losartan for hypertension and atorvastatin for hyperlipidemia. His family history was significant for type 1 diabetes, vitiligo, and lupus in his father; myasthenia gravis in his paternal grandfather; and rheumatoid arthritis in his grandmother. He had no retinopathy or neuropathy, but had prior microalbuminuria with ACR of 45 µg/mg in 2014 followed by normalization. In 2017, albuminuria recurred, with ACR of 912 µg/mg and 1,432 µg/mg on repeat testing. His physical examination was unremarkable. He did not have retinopathy. He was referred to nephrology for further investigation.

Laboratory evaluation revealed HbA_{1c} of 6.5%, creatinine of 0.9 mg/dL, and albumin of 3.8 g/dL. C3, C4, and C-reactive protein levels were normal. Hepatitis B, hepatitis C, HIV, ANA screen, ANCA screen, anti-GBM antibody, anti-DsDNA antibody, Sjogren (SSA, SSB) antibody, anti-Smith antibody, anti-RNP antibody, SPEP and UPEP with IFE, and SCL70 antibody were negative. Urinalysis was positive for 2+ proteinuria and negative for white blood cells, RBCs, squamous epithelial cells, occult blood, nitrites, leukocyte esterase, bilirubin, and ketones. Renal ultrasound was normal.

His serum creatinine remained normal over the ensuing months, but proteinuria continued at 1.4 g/24 h. Because of the rapid progression of his proteinuria despite glycemic control and well-managed hypertension, he underwent a renal biopsy. Pathology showed thickened capillary loops and extensive intramembranous electron–dense deposits with remodeling of the glomerular basement membrane and severe podocyte foot process effacement. Immunofluorescence showed a granular, predominately capillary loop, staining for IgG (3+), C3 (3+), kappa (0-1+), and lambda (0–1+) (Figure 43.1C and D). PLA_2R stain was negative, consistent with membranous glomerulopathy (Figure 43.1C and D), and diabetic kidney disease was not present.

Because of the association between combined variable immunodeficiency and membranous diabetic kidney disease, the patient was referred to immunology. Undetectable IgM was confirmed, but IgA and IgG were normal. Antibody response to the 23-valent pneumococcal vaccine was normal. His renal function remained stable, and proteinuria improved on an angiotensin II receptor blocker.

Patients with type 1 diabetes are at high risk for diabetic kidney disease. We present two patients with well-controlled type 1 diabetes who experienced a dramatic increase in albuminuria and were found to have nondiabetic renal disease (NDRD) on kidney biopsy.

These cases highlight the importance of annual testing of albuminuria and renal function, which is recommended after 5 years of type 1 diabetes and at diagnosis in type 2 diabetes. The risk of diabetic kidney disease occurs in up to 40% of patients with type 1 or type 2 diabetes.[1] Microalbuminuria may be progressive or regress in some patients. NDRD is uncommon but can occur in isolation or with diabetic kidney disease. The etiology of NDRD includes IgA

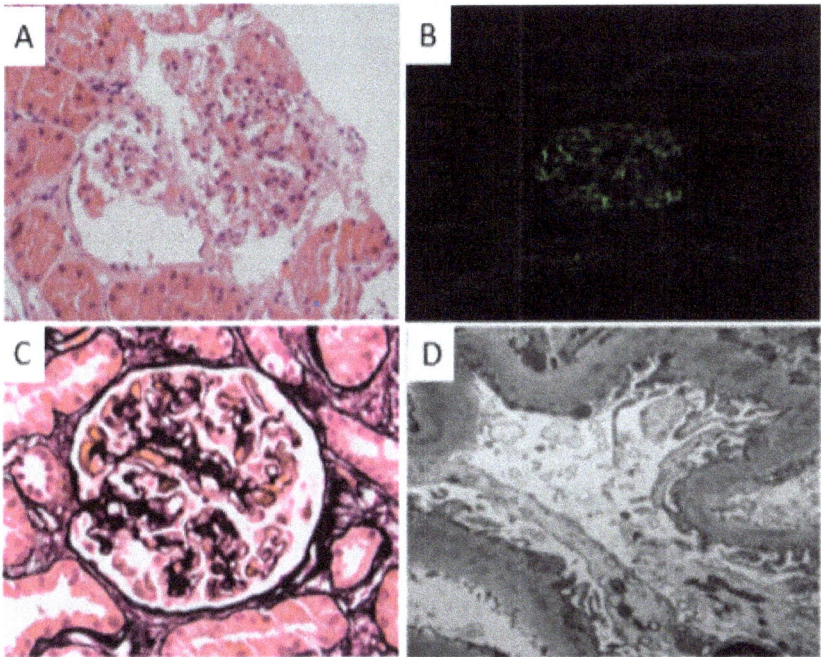

Figure 43.1 — *A*: Light microscopy: mesangial hypercellularity in IgA diabetic kidney disease. *B*: Immunofluorescence microscopy: diffuse mesangial IgA in IgA diabetic kidney disease. *C*: Light microscopy: spikes and pinholes in membranous diabetic kidney disease. *D*: Electron microscopy: electron-dense deposits in subepithelial region in membranous diabetic kidney disease.

diabetic kidney disease, FSGS, crescentic glomerulonephritis, minimal change disease, membranous diabetic kidney disease, and acute interstitial nephritis.[2] In a meta-analysis of subjects with type 2 diabetes, predictors for NDRD include hematuria, absence of retinopathy, shorter diabetes duration, lower HbA$_{1c}$, and lower blood pressure.[3] These results are consistent with results in our patients, neither of whom had retinopathy or neuropathy. Retinopathy is strongly associated with diabetic kidney disease in type 1 diabetes.[4] A study evaluating renal biopsies from subjects with type 1 diabetes found a 12% incidence of NDRD.[2] Patients with type 1 diabetes and NDRD had shorter diabetes duration, with half presenting <5 years, while all subjects with diabetic kidney disease presented after 5 years' duration of type 1 diabetes.[2] Additional predictors of NDRD included absence of neuropathy and presence of proteinuria.[2,5] In both cases presented, a rapid rise in albuminuria triggered the evaluation for NDRD. Both patients had autoimmune or immune deficiency diseases, suggesting the possibility of other etiologies for their proteinuria. The presence of hematuria, along with nephrotic range proteinuria, prompted a renal biopsy in case 1. Despite a completely unremarkable work-up, the rapid rise in albuminuria in case 2 prompted the renal biopsy. Based on existing evidence for NDRD, renal biopsy should be considered in individuals with type 1 diabetes who meet one or more of the following criteria: absence of retinopathy and neuropathy, shorter duration of diabetes, hematuria or RBC casts, rapid progression of renal dysfunction or proteinuria with well-controlled diabetes and hypertension, or risk factors for glomerulopathy.[5]

In conclusion, annual monitoring of renal function and proteinuria is recommended for all patients with type 1 diabetes to test for diabetic kidney disease. Understanding the natural history of diabetic kidney disease and NDRD is crucial to determine when additional work-up, including kidney biopsy, is warranted in patients with changes in albuminuria or kidney function.

COMMENTARY

Almost without exception, proteinuria in patients with diabetes is interpreted as a clinical manifestation of diabetic kidney disease. These two cases remind us that patients with diabetes can and occasionally do develop NDRD. Prevalence of NDRD in type 1 diabetes is lower than in type 2 diabetes, but the overall incidence of NDRD in patients with diabetes is not uncommon. Proteinuria in patients with diabetes with relatively good glycemic control, absence of neuropathy and retinopathy, and sometimes presence of other systemic diseases should alert an astute clinician for the possibility of NDRD. Kidney biopsy confirms the diagnosis.

An important clinical pearl from these two cases is that patients with diabetes and proteinuria may have NDRD, and kidney biopsy is a critical diagnostic tool to identify underlying renal disease in these patients, so proper treatment can be instituted in a timely fashion.

Boris Draznin, MD, PhD

REFERENCES

1. Gross JL, de Azevedo MJ, Silveriro SP, Canani LH, Caramori TZ. Diabetic nephropathy: diagnosis, prevention, and treatment. *Diabetes Care* 2005;28: 164–176

2. Amoah E, Glickman JL, Malchoff CD, Sturgill BC, Kaiser DL, Bolton WK. Clinical identification of nondiabetic renal disease in diabetic patients with type I and type II disease presenting with renal dysfunction. *Am J Nephrol* 1988;8:204–211

3. Liang S, Zhang X-G, Cai G-Y, et al. Identifying parameters to distinguish non-diabetic renal diseases from diabetic nephropathy in patients with type 2 diabetes mellitus: a meta-analysis. *PLoS One* 2013;8:e64184

4. Kramer CK, Retnakaran R. Concordance of retinopathy and nephropathy over time in type 1 diabetes: an analysis of data from the Diabetes Control and Complications Trial. *Diabet Med* 2013;30:1333–1341

5. Teng J, Dwyer KM, Hill P, et al. Spectrum of renal disease in diabetes. *Nephrology* 2014;19:528–536

Case 44

Severe Fetal Malformation Related to Obesity and Type 2 Diabetes

Aswathi Kumar, MD,[1] and Janet B. McGill, MD[1]

The patient was a 33-year-old female who was diagnosed with type 2 diabetes at age 19 years. Her BMI at that age was ~35 kg/m². She initially only required metformin, but stopped taking it and stopped coming to the clinic at age 25 years. She became pregnant at age 28 years and weighed ~298 lb, her BMI had increased to 49 kg/m², and her HbA$_{1c}$ was 9.0%. She started prenatal vitamins after discovering that she was pregnant. Rapid intensification of diabetes therapy ensued, including starting an insulin pump. She was able to attain glucose levels near the target range for pregnancy by about 8 weeks of pregnancy. She had routine ultrasounds, however, at 19 weeks of gestation and the ultrasounds showed that the fetus was likely to be nonviable, with an open cervical neural tube defect (NTD). α-Fetoprotein level was elevated. The pregnancy was terminated despite the patient's religious beliefs, which did not accept abortion.

Testing after the pregnancy showed that the patient was heterozygous for methylenetetrahydrofolate reductase variant A1298C; however, she had normal folate, vitamin B12, and homocysteine levels. Notably, her mother had pernicious anemia and type 2 diabetes.

The patient maintained tight glucose control with the insulin pump, but despite dieting, she was unable to lose weight. At age 30 years, she underwent Roux-en-Y gastric bypass, stopped insulin shortly after surgery, and lost 115 lb in the first 8 months. With guidance from high-risk obstetrics and endocrinology, she became pregnant for the second time. She required metformin and low-dose NPH insulin during the pregnancy and achieved glucose targets without difficulty. Because of her high risk for recurrent NTD, she took 4.0 mg of supplemental folate before and during her second pregnancy. She developed vitamin B12 deficiency during the pregnancy and required parenteral replacement. She also developed atrial fibrillation and was treated with enoxaparin. She delivered a healthy baby boy.

Since delivery, she has remained on metformin 1,000 mg daily and her HbA$_{1c}$ has remained between 5.8 and 6%. She has no known complications of diabetes. She lost a total of 120 lb after bariatric surgery, and weight is now stable. She remains on vitamin supplementation.

[1]Division of Endocrinology, Metabolism, and Lipid Research, Washington University School of Medicine, St. Louis, Missouri

 DOI: 10.2337/9781580407663.44

This case illustrates the risks of pregnancy complicated by diabetes and obesity. Major open NTD in the fetus resulted in termination of the first pregnancy. After bariatric surgery and successful weight loss, along with improved diabetes control, the patient had a subsequent pregnancy with delivery of a healthy baby. The patient followed recommendations for increased folate intake of 4.0 mg daily before and during the pregnancy and for monitoring red blood cell folate and vitamin B12 levels.

Babies of women with diabetes are more likely to have complications, including fetal death, macrosomia, birth injury, and respiratory distress. The National Birth Defects Prevention Study observed a 10-fold increased risk for certain birth defects including holoprosencephaly, longitudinal limb deficiency, heterotaxy, truncus arteriosus, atrioventricular septal defects, and single ventricle complex in offspring of mothers with diabetes. Adequate glycemic control before pregnancy is associated with decreased risk of birth defects.[1]

Independently, obesity is known to cause complications in pregnancy including hypertension and gestational diabetes as well as birth defects. Women who are overweight or obese have a higher risk of having a child with birth defects than women of normal weight. These defects include spina bifida, omphalocele, and heart defects.[2,3] More specifically, epidemiologic data suggest an association between obesity and a range of neural tube defects. A meta-analysis of observational studies evaluating pre- or early pregnancy weight and congenital anomalies showed that obese women were 1.87 times more likely to have a baby affected by any NTD than normal-weight women, and two times as likely to have a pregnancy affected by spina bifida or open NTD.[3] Another meta-analysis also showed that while obesity is associated with a nearly twofold increased risk of NTDs, severe obesity (BMI >38–40 kg/m^2 or weight >110 kg) is associated with a more than three times increased risk for this malformation.[4]

Nutritional deficits due to longstanding poor diet may play a role in the increased risk of birth defects in pregnant women with obesity; however, daily intake of the recommended 400 µg folate did not reduce this risk among women weighing >110 kg, although a 40% risk reduction was seen in women weighing <70 kg.[2] Studies of higher intake of dietary folate found lower risk of NTDs in offspring of obese mothers.[5,6] The Medical Research Council (MRC) study in high-risk women with a prior fetal NTD showed that very high-dose folate supplementation (4.0 mg/day) reduced the risk of recurrent NTD by 72% (relative risk [RR] 0.28, 95% CI 0.12–0.71).[6] Thus, for women at moderate risk of NTD, the recommended dose of supplemental folic acid is 1.0 mg daily, while for women at high risk because of morbid obesity or prior NTD, the recommended dose of folic acid is 4.0 mg daily beginning 3 months before conception.

The risk of having a child with birth defects is increased further in women who are both obese and have diabetes. Obese women with diabetes were 3.1 times more likely to have a baby with a birth defect than normal-weight women without diabetes.[2]

In conclusion, preconception counseling should address the risks of both diabetes and obesity. The added independent risk for neural tube defects in the fetus of a woman with obesity should be discussed, and high doses of folate supplementation should be started 3 months before conception and be continued throughout pregnancy and until breastfeeding has concluded. Achieving a healthy weight is likely to help diabetes control and reduce the added risk that obesity plays in the health of the mother and baby.

COMMENTARY

NTDs are birth defects of the brain, spine, or spinal cord. Spina bifida and anencephaly represent the two most common forms of NTD. These defects happen in the first month of pregnancy, sometimes even before the woman knows she is pregnant, and there is no cure for NTDs.

While the exact causes of NTDs are not known, obesity and poorly controlled diabetes significantly enhance the risk of having a baby with an NTD. It has been strongly suggested that getting enough folic acid before and during pregnancy might prevent most of the NTD.

Among several interesting points of this case is the fact that the patient was heterozygous for methylenetetrahydrofolate reductase variant A1298C, a mutation in the gene of the enzyme that converts folic acid and dietary folate into its active form, L-methylfolate, which is critical in the process of neurotransmitter synthesis. Even though this patient had normal levels of folate, vitamin B12, and homocysteine levels, reduced conversion of folate into L-methylfolate could have contributed to the negative influence of obesity and diabetes.

Weight reduction with Roux-en-Y gastric bypass, better control of diabetes, and supplemental folate before and during her second pregnancy resulted in delivery of a healthy infant. The case highlights the importance of preconception counseling, weight reduction, and glycemic control along with health supplements to avoid birth defects in infants of mothers who are obese and/or have diabetes.

Boris Draznin, MD, PhD

REFERENCES

1. Tinker S, Gilboa S, Moore C, et al. Specific birth defects in pregnancies of women with diabetes: National Birth Defects Prevention Study, 1997–2011. *Am J Obstet Gynecol* 2020;222:176.e1–176.e11

2. Reece A. Obesity, diabetes, and links to congenital defects: a review of the evidence and recommendations for intervention. *J Metarn Fetal Neonatal Med* 2008;21:173–180

3. Stothard K, Tennant P, Bell R, Rankin J. Maternal overweight and obesity and the risk of congenital anomalies. *JAMA* 2009;301:636–650

4. Rasmussen SA, Chu SY, Kim SY, Schmid CH, Lau J. Maternal obesity and risk of neural tube defects: a metaanalysis. *Am J Obstet Gynecol* 2008;198:611–619

5. McMahon DM, Liu J, Zhang H, Torres ME, Best RG. Maternal obesity, folate intake, and neural tube defects in offspring. *Birth Defects Res A Clin Mol Teratol* 2013;97:115–122

6. Prevention of neural tube defects: results of the Medical Research Council Vitamin Study: MRC Vitamin Study Research Group. *Lancet* 1991;338: 131–137

Case 45
Hyperglycemia from Oral Comfort Feeds

Nehu Parimi, MD,[1] Rajani Gundluru, MD,[1] Michael Gardner, MD,[1] and James Sowers, MD[1]

The patient was a 27-year-old male with a complex past medical history of type 1 diabetes since the age 5 years; bipolar, schizoaffective disorder; and polysubstance abuse. He presented with severe diabetic ketoacidosis that developed during an episode of acute opioid withdrawal and was admitted to the medical intensive care unit.

Admission labs showed a blood glucose of 1,290 mg/dL, anion gap of 51, β-hydroxybutyrate of >8 mmol/L, bicarbonate of 9 mmol/L, lactic acid of 8 mmol/L, pH of 7.1, and HbA$_{1c}$ of 11%. He was started on insulin drip for diabetic ketoacidosis and, shortly after admission, was found to have esophageal perforation with left hydropneumothorax, and pneumomediastinum. He underwent emergent left thoracotomy with esophageal resection with spit fistula placement and jejunostomy tube placement for enteral feedings. While ventilated and on continuous feeds, hyperglycemia was controlled on a regimen of basal insulin with NPH or glargine and a correction scale with regular insulin every 4 h with reasonable success.

About 2 months after surgery, the patient began requesting oral comfort items such as hard candy and coffee. These items expanded to include a variety of semi-solids, sweetened beverages, and dairy products. All intake passed into the spit fistula rapidly and initially was disregarded. Intake was unrestricted and eventually reached over 20,000 calories per day, with large amounts of carbohydrate in various forms. Simultaneously, it was noted that his blood glucose levels became more erratic with hyper- and hypoglycemia. It was postulated that oral absorption of carbohydrate from his comfort intake was unpredictably affecting his blood glucose levels.

The patient remained on continuous jejunostomy feedings through most of his 10-month hospitalization, and several insulin regimens were attempted during this time, including a small insulin dose based on the carbohydrate content of his oral comfort intake (in addition to his long-acting insulin used to cover his basal needs and continuous feedings). It appeared that his blood glucose levels fluctuated excessively and correlated somewhat with comfort food intake. Because of behavioral concerns and depletion of food resources on his unit, the patient was placed on a behavioral contract that significantly reduced his access to oral comfort items, although intake was still several quarts per day. After this, his basal insulin requirement

[1]Department of Endocrinology, University of Missouri, Columbia

 DOI: 10.2337/9781580407663.45

declined and blood glucose levels became much less labile. The patient did occasionally have hypoglycemic episodes, usually due to tube feeding disruption, and during some of these episodes, sublingual and buccal administration of glucose or sucrose was given in an attempt to correct hypoglycemia. This attempt was largely unsuccessful. Interestingly, on the rare occasions when his oral comfort intake was interrupted, there was a decline in correctional insulin requirement and even occasional hypoglycemia.

Hypoglycemia is a common problem in hospitalized patient and is usually iatrogenic and correlates with high mortality in severely ill patients.[1] Routinely mild hypoglycemia is treated with 15 g carbohydrate either in the form of glucose tablets, juice, or other high simple-sugar foods. In a meta-analysis of treatment of symptomatic hypoglycemia, patients with diabetes had a higher rate of relief of symptomatic hypoglycemia 15 min after ingestion of glucose tablets when compared to other dietary sugars, such as sucrose and fructose from juice or candy.[2] Another study in 16 healthy volunteers found that liquid sugar or dextrose tablets, but not buccal glucose spray, were effective in increasing plasma glucose within 10 min of ingestion.[3]

In our patient, the isolation of the oral mucosa and proximal esophagus from the rest of the gastrointestinal tract coupled with large intake of carbohydrate-containing liquids and semi-solids provided an interesting setting in which to observe the relative effect of mucosal absorption of carbohydrates on blood glucose levels. The high insulin sensitivity of this patient is proposed to have amplified oscillations in glycemia. The failure of the patient to respond to orally administered corrective carbohydrates during episodes of hypoglycemia poses a paradox not answered by current literature. The implications of this for other patients is a worthy area for investigation, since the evaluation of the oral mucosa as an absorbing surface for organic nutrients has long been neglected.[4] Another area to explore would be the differences in oral absorption of carbohydrates in euglycemic versus hypoglycemic patients.

COMMENTARY

In my view, if one considers diabetes management as a structure that we (providers and patients) build over the years, two basic principles constitute the foundation of this structure. One of them is the diet and another is close follow-up and timely adjustments of medications (especially insulin) to successfully control patients' glycemia.

A patient can "out-eat" any amount of insulin and any medicinal regimen. Reasonable control over the overall caloric intake and the amount of carbohydrate must be instituted. What is reasonable is left to interpretation, but consumption of ~20,000 calories per day is clearly beyond reasonable. Not surprisingly, even high doses of insulin may be ineffective. The danger of using high doses of insulin is evident and becomes an urgent reality when intake is suddenly interrupted while there is "insulin on board." I can share the frustration of his management team when dietary problems are not addressed.

Interruptions in caloric intake are also frequent in patients on tube feeding (enteral nutrition). This explains why many practitioners consider two or three daily injections of NPH insulin more appropriate in such patients than longer-acting insulins. Hospital policy should also include an initiation of intravenous D10 dextrose infusion when enteral nutrition is interrupted for whatever reason.

Why this patient absorbed some food items so efficiently but responded inadequately to sublingual and buccal administration of glucose (when given to correct his hypoglycemia) is unclear. What is clear, however, is that patients in similar situations must be followed very closely and their insulin doses adjusted very frequently.

Boris Draznin, MD, PhD

REFERENCES

1. Fischer KF, Lees JA, Newman JH. Hypoglycemia in hospitalized patients. *N Engl J Med* 1986;315:1245–1250

2. Carlson JN, Schunder-Tatzber S, Neilson CJ, Hood N. Dietary sugars versus glucose tablets for first-aid treatment of symptomatic hypoglycaemia in awake patients with diabetes: a systematic review and meta-analysis. *Emerg Med J* 2017;34:100–106

3. Chlup R, Zapletalova J, Peterson K, et al. Impact of buccal glucose spray, liquid sugars and dextrose tablets on the evolution of plasma glucose concentration in healthy persons. *Biomed Pap Med Fac Univ Palacky Olomouc Czech Repub* 2009;153:205–209

4. Evered DF, Manning AS. The absorption of sugars from the human buccal cavity. *Clin Sci Mol Med* 1976;51:127–132

Case 46

Rethinking Insulin in Type 2 Diabetes

Rebecca J. Morey, MD,[1] and Cynthia Herrick, MD, MPHS[1]

M.B. is a 54-year-old African American woman with a history of type 2 diabetes, sleep apnea on CPAP, hypertension, obesity, and depression. She presented to our clinic for management of her well-controlled type 2 diabetes, which was complicated by neuropathy and microalbuminuria. M.B. was diagnosed with type 2 diabetes at age 44 years and was treated with metformin and insulin. At first meeting she was taking insulin detemir, 38 units daily, and insulin aspart, 15 units three times daily before meals. She reported missing a dose of detemir about once a week and one dose of aspart on most days. She consistently checked her blood glucose levels at least three times daily and reported them to be between 90 and 120 mg/dL. Her C-peptide was 3.92 ng/mL (reference 1.1–4.4 ng/mL) with a blood glucose of 311 mg/dL. Her biggest concern was her obesity, with a BMI of 50 kg/m². She had struggled for decades to successfully lose weight, trying calorie restriction and different fad diets. She reported always feeling hungry. Our initial goal was to assist with weight loss with a secondary goal of simplifying her regimen. At our initial visit, she was started on liraglutide 0.6 mg daily for a week before increasing it to 1.2 mg daily. Her insulin doses were decreased in anticipation of liraglutide taking effect (Table 46.1).

Over the following 6 months she lost 21 lb, going from pant size 2XL to XL. She changed her diet by reducing portions, eliminating fruit juices, and minimizing simple carbohydrates. She stated that, "It just didn't feel that hard; I'm just eating less." She continued to check her blood glucose levels three times daily and felt anxious about stopping. We worked with her to decrease to a single fasting morning blood glucose check over 3 months.

Nine months after initial presentation, she had lost 24 lb from her initial weight, was wearing pant size 16, and remained off insulin. We further simplified her regimen to metformin extended release 750 mg, two tablets once daily with liraglutide 1.8 mg.

She then struggled with significant depression and emotional eating after several deaths in her family. She regained 8 lb; however, even with poor dietary choices, her HbA$_{1c}$ only rose to 6.5%. She was connected with

[1]Division of Endocrinology, Metabolism, and Lipid Research, Washington University School of Medicine, St. Louis, Missouri

DOI: 10.2337/9781580407663.46

Table 46.1—Patient treatment and diabetes data

Time (months)	0	3	6	9	14	18
HbA$_{1c}$ (%)	6.5	6.1	6.2	6.1	6.4	6.5
Weight (lb)	290	277	269.2	266.2	266.8	274.5
Pant size	2X	1X	XL	16–18		
Blood glucose checks per day	4	4	2–3	1	1	1
TDD insulin	83	46	0	0	0	0
Detemir* (daily)	38 units	25 units	—	—	—	—
Aspart* (before meals)	15 units	7 units	—	—	—	—
Metformin extended release*	500 mg t.i.d.	500 mg t.i.d.	500 mg t.i.d.	500 mg b.i.d.	1 g q.a.m.	1.5 g q.a.m.
Liraglutide* (daily)	—	1.2 mg	1.2 mg	1.2 mg	1.8 mg	1.8 mg

*Medications listed are those taken before visit. TDD, total daily dose.

mental health support and was relieved to not worry as much about her diabetes with these additional stressors.

At her initial presentation, this patient had well-controlled glycemia without hypoglycemia and had been on a stable regimen. In these cases, it may be tempting to avoid changes. However, the patient's elevated C-peptide demonstrated that she still had significant endogenous insulin production, and therefore noninsulin options were reasonable. In addition, given her desire for weight loss, reducing insulin use with a glucagon-like peptide-1 receptor agonist (GLP-1RA) was appropriate. Finally, given the patient's multiple comorbidities, the cardiovascular benefits of GLP-1RAs made that class the clear choice.

Liraglutide, 3-mg dose (Saxenda), is approved for weight loss by the U.S. Food and Drug Association. However, insurance coverage is limited, often making it difficult to prescribe. The weight loss benefit of liraglutide is dose dependent. A 2009 *Lancet* study demonstrated mean weight loss of 4.8 kg over 20 weeks (10.5 lb) on 1.8 mg liraglutide.[1] Although 4.8 kg was the mean weight loss, 18.9% of participants lost over 10% of their body weight on this dose. This study suggests that a significant proportion of patients may have robust responses and lose a significant amount of excess body weight.[1] Anecdotally, patients who have difficulty feeling satiated after meals often show the most benefit from GLP-1RA, while patients who eat from boredom or are emotional eaters see less benefit. This patient experienced modest weight regain during a severe depressive episode. However, her glycemic control continued to be excellent, and she remained below her initial weight.

One of the benefits of pursuing noninsulin therapies is reducing the patient's burden of disease. M.B. initially required coaching to stop checking her blood glucose levels after frequently checking them for years. However, once the transition was made, she was able to move from blood glucose checks and insulin four times daily to once-daily medication and monitoring. Ideally, we could have reduced this burden even more by choosing a once-weekly GLP-1RA; however, we were limited by insurance coverage. As the patient's life became busier, she was thankful that she did not need to devote as much energy to managing her diabetes.

GLP-1RAs are increasingly becoming the standard of care for treating type 2 diabetes. One advantage over insulin is the reduction in the risk of hypoglycemia. Additionally, GLP-1RAs are associated with weight loss compared to insulin, which tends to drive weight gain. Data on the three injectable GLP-1RAs available in the U.S. show that they reduce the risk of major adverse cardiovascular events, such as death from cardiovascular disease, nonfatal myocardial infarction, or nonfatal stroke. These benefits are seen most clearly in higher-risk patients.[2–4] By rethinking insulin, patients with type 2 diabetes can benefit from weight loss, simplified dosing regimens, reduced hypoglycemia, and cardiovascular protection.

COMMENTARY

This case study is another great example of the increased and efficacious use of GLP-1RAs in a patient with type 2 diabetes on insulin, with an ultimate goal of removing insulin altogether. Using this class of drugs is especially prudent in patients with obesity and/or atherosclerotic cardiovascular disease. As the authors correctly pointed out, many overweight patients with diabetes lose weight even on lower doses of liraglutide that was approved for weight reduction. Some individuals will not lose that much weight, but the trial is very appropriate. This particular patient lost 24 lb from her original weight, and her HbA_{1c} was 6.5% in the absence of insulin.

Mental well-being is extremely important for successful control of diabetes. Referring this patient to mental health professionals is highly appropriate. One would hope the patient will continue on this path with her diet and therapeutic regimen.

Boris Draznin, MD, PhD

REFERENCES

1. Astrup A, Rossner S, Van Gaal L, et al. Effects of liraglutide in the treatment of obesity: a randomised, double-blind, placebo-controlled study. *Lancet* 2009;374:1606–1616. doi: 10.1016/S0140-6736(09)61375-1

2. Gerstein HC, Colhoun HM, Dagenais GR, et al. Dulaglutide and cardiovascular outcomes in type 2 diabetes (REWIND): a double-blind, randomised placebo-controlled trial. *Lancet* 2019;394:121–130. doi: 10.1016/S0140-6736(19)31149-3

3. Marso SP, Bain SC, Consoli A, et al. Semaglutide and cardiovascular outcomes in patients with type 2 diabetes. *N Engl J Med* 2016;375:1834–1844. doi: 10.1056/NEJMoa1607141

4. Marso SP, Daniels GH, Brown-Frandsen K, et al. Liraglutide and cardiovascular outcomes in type 2 diabetes. *N Engl J Med* 2016;375:311–322. doi: 10.1056/NEJMoa1603827

Case 47

Coincidence or Consequence? A Case of Type 1 Diabetes With Worsening Neuropathy

Cecilia C. Low Wang, MD, FACP[1]

A 28-year-old female with a 23-year history of type 1 diabetes was admitted for diabetic ketoacidosis, precipitated by an upper respiratory infection in the setting of chronic ketosis on a low-carbohydrate diet for the past year. Her serum glucose was 206 mg/dL, bicarbonate was 9 mEq/L, anion gap was 17, and HbA$_{1c}$ was 10.2% on admission. During her hospital stay, the importance of moderate carbohydrate intake with adequate insulin coverage was discussed, and a plan was developed for up-titration of basal insulin after discharge.

She came to the Endocrine clinic to establish care and reported shooting nerve pain in her legs for the past year, more severe at night, worse in her ankles, and more noticeable recently. The pain was sharp, intermittent, up to 8/10 in severity, and improved by stretching and walking. Her blood pressure was 128/84 mmHg, pulse was 91, and BMI 21.4 kg/m^2. She was a well-appearing young woman with normal dorsalis pedis and posterior tibial pulses and no evidence of ulcers, abrasions, or lesions of her feet. Ankle deep tendon reflexes could not be elicited. The sensation in her feet was intact to light touch with a 10-g monofilament. Her basal insulin was continued at 21 units daily in divided doses, as was her rapid-acting insulin with a carbohydrate ratio of 1:10 and correction factor of 1:50 above a blood glucose goal of 100 mg/dL. She was given instructions regarding testing and adjustment of her carbohydrate ratio. She wanted to wait on starting oral medication for her neuropathy, so capsaicin cream was prescribed. Over the next 3 months, she had two visits with a certified diabetes care and education specialist in clinic, and her bolus insulin regimen was further titrated to a final carbohydrate ratio of 1:6 and correction factor of 1:30 >100 mg/dL, with markedly improved glycemic control.

Diabetic neuropathies affect quality of life by causing pain and can cause weakness, ataxia, and increased risk for falls. Two mechanisms have been hypothesized: metabolic abnormalities within the nerve and/or Schwann cells or as another manifestation of diabetic microvascular disease.[1] The diagnosis of diabetic neuropathies is clinical, and nondiabetic causes must be excluded.

[1]University of Colorado School of Medicine, Department of Medicine Division of Endocrinology, Metabolism and Diabetes, Anschutz Medical Campus, Aurora, Colorado

DOI: 10.2337/9781580407663.47

Testing can be done to quantify the type and severity. Progression of diabetic neuropathy is correlated with poor glycemic control. Treatment includes improving glycemic control, addressing symptoms and quality of life, and preventing progression and complications. There is level A evidence for pregabalin, duloxetine, or gabapentin as initial pharmacological treatments for neuropathic pain in diabetes.[2]

Six weeks after her initial appointment, she called to report acute onset of severe itchiness over her right abdomen, which progressed to severe stabbing, shooting, electric pain over her right abdomen ("hot to the touch"), extending around to her mid-back, from her iliac crest up to her axilla, and worsening over time. There was no visible rash at any time. She was preparing for her wedding at the time and was concerned that this would affect wedding and honeymoon plans. She tried a number of nonpharmacological measures and then saw her primary care physician, who felt shingles was unlikely, did laboratory testing to exclude infection or kidney or liver dysfunction, and prescribed gabapentin 100 mg t.i.d., which was up-titrated to 300 mg t.i.d. and provided some relief. Thoracic magnetic resonance imaging (MRI) was unremarkable except for faint hyperintensity from T7 to T10 of unclear significance.

At her Endocrine clinic visit 6 weeks after starting the gabapentin, she reported finally being able to wear some clothing that touched her torso but was still experiencing significant pain, which affected her sleep and daily activities. No focal motor or sensory deficits were detectable on exam. Her HbA$_{1c}$ was 8.2% at the visit. Her gabapentin dose was up-titrated further, and a referral was placed for a neurologist specializing in diabetic neuropathy.

The neurologist's exam revealed decreased sensation to light touch and temperature along the dorsal aspect of the mid forearm and the fourth and fifth digits. Nerve conduction studies showed normal sensory amplitude of the right sural nerve with mildly slowed conduction velocity and normal nerve conduction in the right radial, median, and ulnar sensory nerves and the right peroneal, median, and ulnar motor nerves. Needle electromyography of select muscles of the right C5-T1 myotomes was normal. These findings were consistent with mild sensory polyneuropathy. Her right torso symptoms and thoracic MRI findings were evaluated, but workup was negative.

This patient has a small-fiber neuropathy. Her acute presentation of acute sensory (painful) neuropathy is considered by some to be a distinct variant of distal symmetric polyneuropathy, usually associated with poor glycemic control but may occur after sudden improvement in glycemic control.[3]

The dose of gabapentin was up-titrated to 900 mg t.i.d., which, along with nonpharmacological measures, finally controlled her pain enough to allow her to resume her usual activities 6 months after onset of severe painful neuropathy. At this Endocrine visit, her HbA$_{1c}$ was down to 7.6%. By 2 years after the onset of the acute episode, her dose of gabapentin was successfully tapered to 600 mg q.h.s., which she continues to take currently >5 years after the initial episode.

Treatment-induced neuropathy of diabetes (TIND) has been defined as acute onset of or increase in neuropathic pain and/or autonomic dysfunction within 8 weeks of a substantial decrease in HbA_{1c}. Different mechanisms have been hypothesized including acute epineurial glucose flux,[4] but data are sparse. TIND has been described as a rare complication thought to be due to the rapid improvement in glycemic control and not insulin therapy per se, since it has been reported with oral antihyperglycemic agents and even with fasting. However, a retrospective review of 954 individuals evaluated for possible diabetic neuropathy demonstrated that >10% of patients with an HbA_{1c} reduction >2% over 3 months developed TIND.[5] This patient's HbA_{1c} decreased by 2% over 3 months, and the onset of acute neuropathy occurred <2 months after up-titration of her insulin regimen. It is unknown whether achieving glycemic control more gradually might lower the risk of developing TIND.

COMMENTARY

TIND, which is also known as insulin neuritis, is believed to be a rare small-fiber neuropathy caused by an abrupt improvement in glycemic control in patients with chronic hyperglycemia. At least in one report, most patients with TIND also presented with a rapid progression of retinopathy, which is similarly postulated to be associated with rapid improvement in glycemic control. The severity of TIND may be related to the magnitude of changes in HbA_{1c}, as well as in the rate of this improvement of glycemic control. It is possible that some patients may also exhibit deterioration of diabetic kidney disease as well, pointing out the relationship between the rapid improvement of glycemia and microvascular disease.

Even though these situations are rare, it might be reasonable to limit decreases in HbA_{1c} in the course of glycemic management of diabetes to <2% per 3 months.

Boris Draznin, MD, PhD

REFERENCES

1. Barrett EJ, Liu Z, Khamaisi M, et al. Diabetic microvascular disease: an Endocrine Society scientific statement. *J Clin Endocrinol Metab* 2017;102:4343–4410. doi: 10.1210/jc.2017-01922

2. American Diabetes Association. 11. Microvascular complications and foot care: *Standards of Medical Care in Diabetes—2020. Diabetes Care* 2020;43(Suppl. 1): S135–S151. https://doi.org/10.2337/dc20-s011

3. Oyibo SO, Prasad YDM, Jackson NJ, Jude EB, Boulton AJM. The relationship between blood glucose excursions and painful diabetic peripheral neuropathy: a pilot study. *Diabet Med* 2002;19:870–873

4. Low PA, Singer W. Treatment-induced neuropathy of diabetes: an energy crisis? *Brain* 2015;138:2–10

5. Gibbons CH, Freeman R. Treatment-induced neuropathy of diabetes: an acute, iatrogenic complication of diabetes. *Brain* 2015;138:43–52. https://doi.org/10.1093/brain/awu307

Case 48

Challenges to the Management of Diabetes in Patients Who Undergo Ventricular Assist Device (VAD) Implantation

Chinenye O. Usoh, MD,[1] Donald A. McClain, MD, PhD,[1] and Barbara A. Pisani, DO[2]

A 74-year-old man with a history of ischemic cardiomyopathy (ejection fraction 30%), atrial fibrillation, obstructive sleep apnea, type 2 diabetes complicated by peripheral neuropathy, diabetic foot ulcer, retinopathy, and stage 3 chronic kidney disease (CKD) presented to the heart failure clinic for evaluation of heart failure refractory to diuretic therapy. At initial consultation, he reported taking 60 units daily of concentrated insulin glargine. Diabetes had been diagnosed at least 20 years prior and was managed by his primary care provider. He had a strong family history of diabetes in his mother and two brothers. His HbA_{1c} was 9.7%. The patient was noted to be severely volume-overloaded in clinic. Hospital admission for intravenous diuresis was recommended in the setting of CKD. During this hospitalization, the glucose management team (GMT) was consulted, and the patient was subsequently discharged on glargine 30 units nightly and lispro 10 units before meals. He was evaluated for ventricular assist device (VAD) and underwent implantation 4 months after initial consultation. About 1 month after VAD implant, he was again admitted for management and evaluation of low flow/speed alarms on VAD. GMT was consulted for overnight hypoglycemia on the above regimen. Creatinine was noted to have improved from baseline. Glargine was decreased to 20 units nightly and mealtime lispro was discontinued. Four months after VAD implant, his HbA_{1c} was 6.4% and has remained in this range for the past year.

There are many challenges to the management of diabetes in the typical clinic patient. However, management of diabetes in patients with heart failure is particularly challenging. This case highlights the unique obstacles that arise and guidance on the management of diabetes in patients undergoing VAD implantation.

The major cause of death for individuals with diabetes is cardiovascular disease. The prevalence of heart failure in people with diabetes (10–20%) is about fourfold higher than in the general population, and conversely it is estimated that 20–40% of patients with heart failure have diabetes.[1] Diabetes leads to

[1]Endocrinology and Metabolism Section. [2]Cardiovascular Medicine Section, Department of Internal Medicine, Wake Forest University School of Medicine, Winston-Salem, North Carolina.

DOI: 10.2337/9781580407663.48

functional and morphological abnormalities within the heart. Individuals with diabetes have evidence of left ventricular remodeling, specifically increased left ventricular mass, and dilation leading to systolic and diastolic dysfunction.[2] In cases of refractory heart failure, a heart transplant may be needed. With the limited availability of donor hearts, VADs are being used more as either a bridge to transplantation or destination therapy.

Potential complications after VAD implantation include neurological dysfunction/stroke, pump thrombosis, gastrointestinal bleed, renal dysfunction, and infection. Individuals with diabetes already have a higher risk of these issues compared to people without diabetes. Studies have also shown a higher risk of death after VAD implantation in patients with type 2 diabetes.[3,4] There have also been reports of decreased insulin requirements after VAD implantation.[5] It is hypothesized that this could be due to decreased inflammation, improved perfusion, and improved lifestyle. Management of diabetes is already multifaceted, and no patients are exactly the same. Heart failure and VAD implant increases that complexity.

Our patient was hospitalized, so close monitoring of blood glucose levels was feasible and appropriate recommendations for insulin could be made. It is important for providers to be aware of potential changes in insulin requirements after VAD implantation. Another challenge is that postoperative courses after implant may vary significantly for patients. VAD implantation is sometimes complicated by infections (such as driveline or surgical site) in 20–30% of cases and can also lead to renal dysfunction and thrombosis resulting in stroke and neurological dysfunction in the months after implantation, all of which can complicate glycemic management. Many patients are motivated to change their lifestyle to reduce their risk of these complications. Activity levels generally increase and exercise is better tolerated because of the improved tissue perfusion and improved pulmonary function. However, there are still many individuals who do not alter poor dietary and exercise habits and have worsening control of diabetes,[5] resulting in poor outcomes. A diabetes regimen should be tailored to the individual, and a healthy lifestyle should be promoted at each visit and every opportunity. A potential solution to the patient variability is the use of continuous glucose monitoring (CGM). Having the patient wear a CGM in the weeks to months after VAD implantation allows for close monitoring and quick adjustments to the diabetes regimen.

In conclusion, changes in insulin requirements are often seen after VAD implantation. Each patient is unique, and the diabetes regimen should be tailored to the individual patient. Providers should be aware of these issues and potentially use technology such as CGM for close monitoring after implantation.

COMMENTARY

Treatment of patients with diabetes and congestive heart failure represents significant challenges. Unfortunately, the number of these patients has increased in the last decade as heart failure has emerged as one of the frequent cardiovascular complications of diabetes. While treatment of heart failure remains beyond the scope of this volume, management of diabetes in these patients falls firmly into the sphere of competency of diabetologists.

This particular case deals with a specific aspect of therapy, addressing challenges of VAD implantation. As with any other aspect of diabetes management, close follow-up and timely adjustments in insulin therapy are key for successful glycemic control. Most certainly, CGM would be of immense help to his management team.

In the patient in this case, insulin requirement decreased significantly, resulting in a lower dose of glargine and discontinuation of mealtime insulin. With these changes, patient's HbA_{1c} came down to 6.4% after VAD implant and remained at this level for the past year.

Boris Draznin, MD, PhD

REFERENCES

1. Dei Cas A, Khan SS, Butler J, et al. Impact of diabetes on epidemiology, treatment, and outcomes of patients with heart failure. *JACC Heart Fail* 2015;3: 136–145. 2015/02/11. doi: 10.1016/j.jchf.2014.08.004

2. Dhingra R, Vasan RS. Diabetes and the risk of heart failure. *Heart Fail Clin* 2012;8:125–133. doi: 10.1016/j.hfc.2011.08.008

3. Usoh CO, Sherazi S, Szepietowska B, et al. Influence of diabetes mellitus on outcomes in patients after left ventricular assist device implantation. *Ann Thorac Surg* 2018;106:555–560. doi: 10.1016/j.athoracsur.2018.02.045

4. Butler J, Howser R, Portner PM, et al. Diabetes and outcomes after left ventricular assist device placement. *J Card Fail* 2005;11:510–515. doi: 10.1016/j.cardfail.2005.05.003

5. Choudhary N, Chen L, Kotyra L, et al. Improvement in glycemic control after left ventricular assist device implantation in advanced heart failure patients with diabetes mellitus. *ASAIO J* 2014;60:675–680. doi: 10.1097/MAT.0000000000000127

Insulin and Heroin: An Unfortunate Mix in an Overlooked Population

Amro Ilaiwy, MD,[1] Jennifer V. Rowell, MD,[1] and Beatrice D. Hong, MD[1]

A 35-year-old woman was evaluated in the emergency department after she was found unconscious at home. Her medical history included type 1 diabetes diagnosed at the age of 10 years and managed with a Medtronic G670 insulin pump and Dexcom G6 continuous glucose monitor. She also had a known history of intravenous drug abuse. Police conducted a home welfare check when the patient did not show up to work. She was found confused and surrounded by spoons, syringes filled with heroin, subcutaneous insulin needles, and insulin pump infusion sets and continuous glucose monitoring (CGM) transmitter and inserters. Laboratory evaluation on admission revealed the following:

Blood glucose: 1,095 mg/dL
β-Hydroxybutyrate: >8 mg/dL
Arterial blood pH: 6.95
Bicarbonate: 7 mEq/L
Potassium: 6 mEq/L
Anion gap: 33
Lactate, venous: 8.7 mg/dL
Creatinine: 3.2 mg/dL (baseline creatinine: 0.6 mg/dL)
HbA$_{1c}$: 7.6%

To treat the diabetic ketoacidosis and hyperkalemia, aggressive hydration with intravenous fluids and insulin drip were initiated, resulting in significant clinical and laboratory improvement. The patient's mental status improved with resolution of acidosis and she was able to provide her own history. The patient identified malfunction of her insulin pump as the cause of her admission. Subcutaneous insulin injections dosed per her off-pump plan failed, resulting in acidosis and coma. The addition of opioids further potentiated kidney injury and metabolic disturbances. Interestingly, her HbA$_{1c}$ was 7.6%, indicating acceptable glycemic control despite her chronic struggles with polysubstance abuse. The patient had a background in health

[1]Division of Endocrinology, Department of Medicine, Duke University Medical Center, Durham, North Carolina

 DOI: 10.2337/9781580407663.49

care and was observed to have a high level of health literacy. During hospitalization, she was transitioned off insulin drip and back to the Medtronic G670 pump, with excellent inpatient glycemic control. After using a multidisciplinary team of pain specialists, internists, and endocrinologists, she improved and was subsequently discharged home.

During her admission, the patient shared remarkable and meticulous observations on being a functioning heroin addict living with type 1 diabetes. She noticed that her daily requirements of both basal and prandial insulin were significantly lower on days when actively using heroin compared to days she abstained from use. This phenomenon was observed during the acute use of heroin independent of carbohydrate intake and stood true even when she consumed a fixed amount of carbohydrates. Based on this observation, she set up two different basal insulin profiles: one for days when she was "clean" and another for days when she was using heroin, with a 20% reduction in basal insulin requirements implemented in the latter. She also increased her insulin-to-carbohydrate ratio while using heroin to overcome the decrease in prandial insulin needs.

The mechanism by which opioids affect glycemic control is complex and poorly understood. A case study of patients in the U.K. between 1998 and 2012 first linked tramadol to an increased risk of hospitalization due to hypoglycemia when compared to codeine.[1] While tramadol was specifically identified, later studies suggested this phenomenon could be due to a class effect. In a small clinical trial, Carey et al.[2] elucidated the effect of morphine infusion over 2 h compared to normal saline infusion. Morphine infusion led to an ~30% reduction in plasma epinephrine with reduced endogenous glucose production and attenuation of symptoms induced by hypoglycemia. This study was the first to define the concept of hypoglycemia-associated autonomic failure induced by opioids and to suggest some utility in identifying this phenomenon when considering safer intensive glycemic control in diabetes.[2]

This case highlights the need to consider the insulin-sensitizing role of opioids,[3] and consideration should be given towards making insulin dose adjustments in patients with type 1 diabetes during periods of recreational opioid use. This overlooked issue is also highly relevant in the aging population of patients with diabetes treated with high doses of prescription opioids. It is important to note that patients treated with prescription opioids for chronic pain tend to be older and have higher rates of adverse events due to multiple comorbidities.[4] Larger-scale studies are needed to address the impact of opioids on glycemic control in this overlooked population.

COMMENTARY

The main point of this case is how little we know about the influence of substance abuse on the course and management of diabetes. While most of us would prefer that this never happens, the reality of life is different, and patients with diabetes take or abuse either illicit or prescription medications. The substances involved may be in a form of cannabis, hallucinogens, opioids, and stimulants.

Certainly, patients with diabetes may take opioids to manage diabetes-related and non–diabetes-related pain, especially neuropathic and musculoskeletal. The effect of opioids and other illicit drugs on blood glucose levels in patients with diabetes may be significant. But even more significant is that drug abuse is likely to lead to behavioral changes that are detrimental to good glycemic control. Patients lose control over their action, lie to providers and family members, ignore therapeutic recommendation, and skip follow-up. Even patients with high health literacy and good general (or even medical) education are not immune from these lapses in judgement and behavior.

In this particular case, opioids seemed to reduce the patient's glycemia, so she adjusted insulin on the days of taking these drugs. In some patients, the effect of opioids might be opposite or may have no impact on glycemic control. In any event, abuse of illicit or prescription drugs will more likely than not lead to substantial difficulties in treating patients with diabetes.

Boris Draznin, MD, PhD

REFERENCES

1. Fournier JP, Azoulay L, Yin H, Montastruc JL, Suissa S. Tramadol use and the risk of hospitalization for hypoglycemia in patients with noncancer pain. *JAMA Intern Med* 2015;175:186–193

2. Carey M, Gospin R, Goyal A, et al. Opioid receptor activation impairs hypoglycemic counterregulation in humans. *Diabetes* 2017;66:2764–2773

3. Fruzzetti F, Bersi C, Parrini D, Ricci C, Genazzani AR. Effect of long-term naltrexone treatment on endocrine profile, clinical features, and insulin sensitivity in obese women with polycystic ovary syndrome. Fertil Steril 2002;77:936–944

4. Sterling V. Special considerations for opioid use in elderly patients with chronic pain. *US Pharm* 2018;43:26–30

Index